"Wise, hopeful, funny, and in___ mys-
teries of eating disorder treatme___ sense
out of the confusion as she guide___ ___aling.
I wish my family and I could have read this book during my struggle with
anorexia and bulimia. This is a must-read!"

—Jenni Schaefer, author of Life Without Ed: How One Woman Declared
Independence from Her Eating Disorder and How You Can Too

"In this well-written and readable book, Carrie Arnold guides the adolescent with an eating disorder through what to expect in the recovery
process using her own often-bumpy recovery as illustration. Providing tips
for everyday survival in the real world and a broader view to help stay the
course to health, her message is a powerful and encouraging one, made all
the more believable to the adolescent sufferer because she has been there.
Carrie also provides information on internal thoughts of the eating disorder that can help parents gain insight into what their adolescent is experiencing and how they might respond."

*—Kathleen A. Mammel, M.D., Chief, Adolescent Pediatrics,
William Beaumont Hospital, and Clinical Assistant Professor
of Pediatrics, Wayne State University*

"Humor and stark honesty are Arnold's trademarks. Most writers un-
critically throw in everything that has ever been said of eating disorders;
Arnold pares it down to up-to-date and accessible science. This book is a
wonderful combination of wit and wisdom."

—Laura Collins, author of Eating with Your Anorexic

"This book is an insightful account of one person's struggle with an eating
disorder. It offers a helpful mix of information, ranging from the personal
to the professional. I expect this book will be helpful to young adults with
an eating disorder *and* their families."

*—Daniel le Grange, Ph.D., Associate Professor of Psychiatry and Director,
Eating Disorders Program at The University of Chicago*

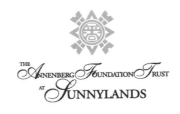

THE ANNENBERG FOUNDATION TRUST AT SUNNYLANDS

The Annenberg Foundation Trust at Sunnylands'
Adolescent Mental Health Initiative

Patrick E. Jamieson, Ph.D., *series editor*

In addition to *Next to Nothing*, other books in this
series for young people are planned on the following topics:

Bipolar Disorder (2006)—now available:
*Mind Race: A Firsthand Account of One Teenager's
Experience With Bipolar Disorder,*
by Patrick E. Jamieson, Ph.D., with Moira A. Rynn, M.D.

Depression (2007)—now available:
*Monochrome Days: A Firsthand Account of One Teenager's
Experience With Depression,*
by Cait Irwin, with Dwight L. Evans, M.D., and Linda Wasmer Andrews

Social Anxiety Disorder (2007)—now available:
*What You Must Think of Me: A Firsthand Account of One
Teenager's Experience With Social Anxiety Disorder,*
by Emily Ford, with Michael Liebowitz, M.D., and Linda Wasmer Andrews

Schizophrenia (2007)
*Me, Myself, and Them: A Firsthand Account of One Young Person's
Experience With Schizophrenia,*
by Kurt Snyder, with Raquel E. Gur, M.D., Ph.D., and Linda Wasmer Andrews

Obsessive-Compulsive Disorder (2008)
*The Thought that Counts: A Firsthand Account of One Teenager's Experience With
Obsessive-Compulsive Disorder,* by Jared Douglas Kant, with Martin Franklin, Ph.D.,
and Linda Wasmer Andrews

Substance Abuse (2008)
*Chasing the High: A Firsthand Account of One Young Person's Experience With
Substance Abuse,* by Kyle Keegan, with Howard B. Moss, M.D., and Beryl Lieff Benderly

Suicide Prevention (2008)
Eight Stories Up: An Adolescent Chooses Hope Over Suicide,
by DeQuincy A. Lezine, Ph.D., with David Brent, M.D.

Also available in the series for parents and other adults:

If Your Adolescent Has Depression or Bipolar Disorder (2005)
Dwight L. Evans, M.D., and Linda Wasmer Andrews

If Your Adolescent Has an Eating Disorder (2005)
B. Timothy Walsh, M.D., and V. L. Cameron

If Your Adolescent Has an Anxiety Disorder (2006)
Edna B. Foa, Ph.D., and Linda Wasmer Andrews

If Your Adolescent Has Schizophrenia (2006)
Raquel E. Gur, M.D., Ph.D., and Ann Braden Johnson, Ph.D.

Next to Nothing

*A Firsthand Account of
One Teenager's Experience
With an Eating Disorder*

Carrie Arnold

with B. Timothy Walsh, M.D.

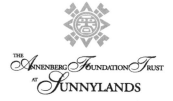

THE ANNENBERG FOUNDATION TRUST
AT SUNNYLANDS

The Annenberg Foundation Trust at Sunnylands'
Adolescent Mental Health Initiative

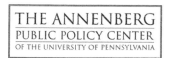

THE ANNENBERG
PUBLIC POLICY CENTER
OF THE UNIVERSITY OF PENNSYLVANIA

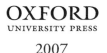

OXFORD
UNIVERSITY PRESS

2007

OXFORD
UNIVERSITY PRESS

Oxford University Press, Inc., publishes works that further
Oxford University's objective of excellence
in research, scholarship, and education.

The Annenberg Foundation Trust at Sunnylands
The Annenberg Public Policy Center of the University of Pennsylvania
Oxford University Press

Oxford   New York
Auckland   Cape Town   Dar es Salaam   Hong Kong   Karachi
Kuala Lumpur   Madrid   Melbourne   Mexico City   Nairobi
New Delhi   Shanghai   Taipei   Toronto

With offices in
Argentina   Austria   Brazil   Chile   Czech Republic   France   Greece
Guatemala   Hungary   Italy   Japan   Poland   Portugal   Singapore
South Korea   Switzerland   Thailand   Turkey   Ukraine   Vietnam

Library of Congress Cataloging-in-Publication Data
Arnold, Carrie, 1980–
Next to nothing : a firsthand account of one teenager's experience with an eating disorder /
by Carrie Arnold with B. Timothy Walsh.
    p. cm.—(Annenberg Foundation Trust at Sunnylands' adolescent mental
health initiative)
"The Annenberg Foundation Trust at Sunnylands, the Annenberg Public Policy Center."
Includes bibliographical references and index.
ISBN 978-0-19-530965-2; 978-0-19-530966-9 (pbk.)
1. Arnold, Carrie, 1980—Mental health.   2. Eating disorders in adolescence—Patients—
Biography.   3. Eating disorders—Treatment.   I. Walsh, B. Timothy, 1946–   II. Title.
RJ506.E18A76 2007
618.92'85260092—dc22   [B]   2007004753

9 8 7 6 5 4 3 2 1

Printed in the United States of America
on acid-free paper

Contents

Foreword

The Adolescent Mental Health Initiative (AMHI) was created by The Annenberg Foundation Trust at Sunnylands to share with mental health professionals, parents, and adolescents the advances in treatment and prevention now available to adolescents with mental health disorders. The Initiative was made possible by the generosity and vision of Ambassadors Walter and Leonore Annenberg, and the project was administered through the Annenberg Public Policy Center of the University of Pennsylvania in partnership with Oxford University Press.

The Initiative began in 2003 with the convening, in Philadelphia and New York, of seven scholarly commissions made up of over 150 leading psychiatrists and psychologists from around the country. Chaired by Drs. Edna B. Foa, Dwight L. Evans, B. Timothy Walsh, Martin E. P. Seligman, Raquel E. Gur, Charles P. O'Brien, and Herbert Hendin, these commissions were tasked with assessing the state of scientific research on the prevalent mental disorders whose onset occurs predominantly between the ages of 10 and 22. Their collective

findings now appear in a book for mental health professionals and policy makers titled *Treating and Preventing Adolescent Mental Health Disorders* (2005). As the first product
of the Initiative, that book also identified a research agenda
that would best advance our ability to prevent and treat
these disorders, among them anxiety disorders, depression
and bipolar disorder, eating disorders, substance abuse, and
schizophrenia.

The second prong of the Initiative's three-part effort is a
series of smaller books for general readers. Some of the books
are designed primarily for parents of adolescents with a specific
mental health disorder. And some, including this one, are
aimed at adolescents themselves who are struggling with a
mental illness. All of the books draw their scientific information in part from the AMHI professional volume, presenting it
in a manner that is accessible to general readers of different
ages. The "teen books" also feature the real-life story of one
young person who has struggled with—and now manages—a
given mental illness. They serve as both a source of solid research about the illness and as a roadmap to recovery for
afflicted young people. Thus they offer a unique combination
of medical science and firsthand practical wisdom in an effort to inspire adolescents to take an active role in their own
recovery.

The third part of the Sunnylands Adolescent Mental
Health Initiative consists of two Web sites. The first, www.
CopeCareDeal.org, addresses teens. The second, www.oup.
com/us/teenmentalhealth, provides updates to the medical
community on matters discussed in *Treating and Preventing
Adolescent Mental Health Disorders*, the AMHI professional
book.

We hope that you find this volume, as one of the fruits of the Initiative, to be helpful and enlightening.

Patrick Jamieson, Ph.D.
Series Editor
Adolescent Risk Communication Institute
Annenberg Public Policy Center
University of Pennsylvania
Philadelphia, PA

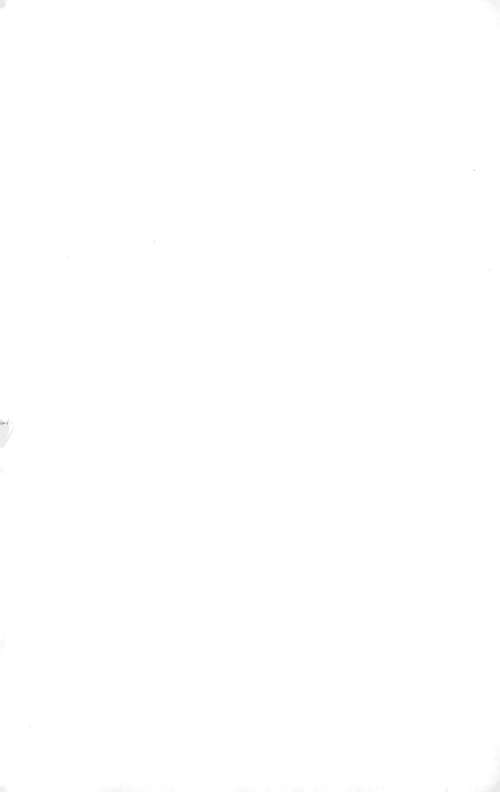

Preface

As I began my long decent into anorexia and bulimia almost eight years ago, I found plenty of reading material on what it was like to be ill, and stories of people who had recovered. But I found virtually nothing describing a young person's actual experience of an eating disorder, nor a practical guide on how to navigate my way through the tumultuous terrain of treatment and recovery. *Next to Nothing* fills the gap between self-discovery and self-help.

The title of this book—*Next to Nothing*—was suggested by my editor Sarah Harrington, and it perfectly describes my experiences with an eating disorder. It captures the sense of despair I felt as the eating disorder took over my life and left me with nothing besides the rituals it ruthlessly demanded. I was nothing if I was not perfect, and I could not be perfect until I had starved myself down to nothing. I had to eat the perfect foods, and next to nothing fit the bill. I had to have the perfect exercise routine, which left me with next to nothing else to do. And finally, as I entered recovery, I found I had next to nothing left in my life, due to the years and years I had devoted to my eating disorder.

In those moments of extreme despair, when I found myself engaging in bizarre food-related behaviors that I did not understand but felt compelled to do—cooking seven-course meals only to chuck them in the trash bin, or frantically sucking down vast quantities of sweets at 2 A.M., purging, and then collapsing into a deep sleep—I felt a profound sense of shame and isolation. I was crazy. I was a freak. No one would ever understand. Out of this experience I wrote my first book, a memoir titled *Running on Empty*, and I have also included my personal experiences with anorexia and bulimia in that book.

For this book I have teamed up with Dr. B. Timothy Walsh, director of the Eating Disorders Research Unit at the New York State Psychiatric Institute. Dr. Walsh is also a professor in the Department of Psychiatry at Columbia University's College of Physicians and Surgeons, and a past president of the Academy for Eating Disorders. In 2003, Dr. Walsh chaired a distinguished professional commission on adolescent eating disorders. This commission was convened by the Annenberg Foundation Trust at Sunnylands as part of a larger initiative to enhance our understanding of mental health disorders in young people. Much of the scientific information in this book comes from a report issued by the Annenberg commission. By combining my personal experiences with Dr. Walsh's professional expertise, this book helps you look at eating disorders from every angle. With Dr. Walsh's assistance, I have provided information on the origins and medical consequences of eating disorders, as well as advice on how to find treatment and maintain your own recovery.

These are not step-by-step instructions—everyone's eating disorder is slightly different, and everyone's recovery will be, too. I have included my own first-person experiences both to provide comfort and reassurance that you are not alone in your struggles, and also to include some of the recovery strategies that have worked for me. However, let me provide a word of caution: The advice and knowledge contained within these pages is no substitute for professional guidance. This book is meant to be a starting point, a compass of sorts. A team of qualified professionals, such as a therapist, a dietician, a pediatrician or medical doctor, and/or a psychiatrist, will provide you with the map.

Though *Next to Nothing* was written primarily as a resource for young people, I hope that their loved ones, such as parents, siblings, relatives, friends, and other concerned adults will benefit from the information contained within. My story may be quite different from that of your loved one's, but even just a glimpse into their experience may be of use to you.

I offer my story not just as a warning of how far you can fall, but as a reminder of the hope that remains when you climb back up. Eating disorders are treatable, even curable, and new therapies are being devised and tested every day. If you read no further in this book, know this: There is hope. As long as you breathe, there is always hope. A happy, fulfilling life awaits you on the other side of an eating disorder. I hope to see you there.

If you read no further in this book, know this: There is hope.

Next to Nothing

Chapter One

A Very Heavy Weight: Life With Anorexia and Bulimia

F or almost seven years, I lived a double life.

On the outside, I was intelligent, happy, successful. I was valedictorian in high school, and at the top of my class in college. I was well-liked by friends, family, and professors. To everyone, it seemed, I had it all together.

What troubled me, though, was what people couldn't see: the hours spent poring over calorie-counting guides, how I wore out countless pairs of gym shoes on the treadmill, the constant adding and subtracting calories and fat grams in my head so I would never eat more than I "should," and going for days without eating a thing only to binge wildly as my famished body overrode all my mental demands to starve.

I never intended to be sick, or even wanted to be sick. I thought that losing weight would make me perfect. I thought it would make me happy.

I wound up being more miserable than I ever dreamed possible.

I was suffering from an eating disorder.

Consumed by ED

Eating disorders are cunning diseases. They creep up on you. They make you think that starving, binge eating, and purging are the answers to your problems. Then they become problems in and of themselves. They wind up consuming you whole. They will kill you, if you let them. I almost let them. After seven long years of fighting, after countless hours of therapy, several hospitalizations, long-term residential treatment, and physical and emotional heartache both for myself and for all those who dared to stand by me, I can finally say that I have made it to the other side. I'm not cured; I'm not perfect. My eating disorder (whom I've named Ed, from the acronym ED, Eating Disorder) still occasionally informs me that my butt is too fat.

To which I say, "Ed, if you don't like the size of my butt, you can just go kiss it."

I believed, for the longest time, that my behaviors were perfectly normal and healthy. No one ever told me about the dangers of dieting and overexercise. No one told me that even occasional purging can kill. No one told me that laxatives were ruthlessly addictive and could cause bowel problems for years down the road. What *did* people tell me? How good I looked as I lost weight. How self-disciplined I must be for always going to the gym or never eating dessert. Or how lucky I was to be so thin that I could eat anything I wanted.

I wanted to smack them.

It's hard to remember, in a culture that encourages and glorifies thinness, that eating disorders are real, diagnosable psychiatric illnesses. Magazine articles and television specials tend to gloss over the more realistic parts of eating disorders: the social isolation, the complete physical weakness and exhaustion, the multitude of physical side effects, and the long, winding road back to "normal." You are not starving and binge eating and purging because you are strong; you are engaged in these behaviors because you are sick. Yet if one is thin, we are told, all will be well. I was never thin enough to appease my eating disorder. Not when I was told I was dying, not when I was hospitalized three times, not when I couldn't even sit in a chair without hurting because I was

I was never thin enough to appease my eating disorder.

so thin. I was simply and utterly dominated by my illness.

There was a voice in my head (the one I named Ed) who told me all sorts of things. He told me what to eat and when, what exercises were the best for burning calories, and what lies to tell to my parents when they asked me what I ate or how much I weighed. He also never forgot to remind me how fat I really was. Keep in mind, I was never psychotic—I knew that this voice originated within me. Neither was I possessed by the devil (not in a literal sense, anyway).

Let me put it this way: We all carry on a dialogue with ourselves. We all have thoughts in our heads, mostly benign, that say "Pull up your socks—you're getting a blister on your heel" or "That man is a terrible driver." However, when you suffer from an eating disorder, that voice instead says things like, "You're fat," "You're worthless," "Don't eat that!" or "Look how much self-control you have when you don't eat."

Ed and I occupied one mind and one body for many years. I had a bout of borderline anorexia at the age of 12. Though I temporarily pulled myself out of it, Ed never truly left me alone, causing an extreme perfectionism that was brutal on my self-esteem. At school, when I got 98 out of 100 questions right on a test, he asked me why I had to go and mess up the other two answers. He told me I would never get into college. When I did, he said I would never succeed. Ed also played games and compared my body with every person that I passed at school or on the street. If I was heavier, then I was a failure—even if the other person was a seven-year-old girl.

As I went off to college in western Michigan, my eating disorder pounced on my anxieties and insecurities about school. Watching every morsel of food that I put in my mouth and constantly trekking over to the gym for a workout gave me a feeling of accomplishment that I was unable to achieve as a freshman in sophomore-level classes. The eating disorder also proved a consolation for having few friends—if I didn't have friends, I would have more time to work out and study.

Obsessing About Food

The more time I spent with my eating disorder, the more my thoughts centered on food. When to get it, when to get rid of it, how to avoid it. I fantasized about rich desserts. I also fantasized about lettuce. As malnutrition set in, I started to *dream* about food, my pillow damp with drool when I awoke in the morning. I missed freeway exits because I was analyzing the calories and fat grams in my sugar-free yogurt (or apple, or carrot sticks). These thoughts totally and utterly preoccupied me.

When I was restricting, I would spend hours in the grocery store, staring at food labels, checking to make sure that the foods I would purchase had acceptably low amounts of calories, fat, sodium, fiber, and cholesterol. Precious few foods did. I panicked at the thought of eating with other people, or eating food I hadn't personally prepared, or going over my acceptable caloric limits for the day, or any number of situations that usually accompany eating. I pored over cookbooks, ogling pictures of rich desserts that I could no longer imagine eating, trying in vain to scratch the pictures and elicit a smell. I would make myself walk the longest route to anywhere in order to burn more calories.

As anorexia and starvation firmly took hold of my brain, my behavior became even more bizarre. I watched cooking programs in every spare moment, even while running on the treadmill. I reorganized my pantries so that all I could see on the packages of food were the labels. I weighed myself several times a day on several different scales so that I could make *absolutely sure* I wasn't gaining weight. My "meals" of carrot sticks and mustard instead became mustard and carrot sticks. And, just as the Eskimos had almost a hundred different words for "snow," I developed numerous names for "hunger." There was the pleasant variety, just intruding enough to let me know I was losing weight—the hunger that prompted me to go crack open another diet soda. Next was the gnawing variety, usually characterized by the telltale growl of the stomach. Lastly, there was the insane variety, the claw-out-your-eyeballs-with-need hunger, the kind where my stomach seemed like a vacuum, sucking in every internal organ in order to feed its voracious appetite.

My "meals" of carrot sticks and mustard instead became mustard and carrot sticks.

When I was engaged in bulimic behaviors, I spent all of my time planning my next binge and purge. I went out in howling blizzards to purchase binge food. I nearly bankrupted myself buying laxatives and diet pills. I knew which supermarkets had apathetic cashiers or self-checkout lanes so that I wouldn't get weird stares for buying a cart full of Krispy Kremes and Ex-Lax. I would only eat at restaurants where I knew I could purge in secret. As the disorder deepened, I became utterly paranoid that someone would discover my dirty little secret, and I found a million little tricks to prevent people from smelling the vomit on my breath or the mess in the toilet.

My entire day became demarcated by bulimia: when I would binge, where I would purge. The all-consuming frenzy that went into planning a binge, buying the food, sucking it all down. The horror at realizing I had eaten *everything* in my apartment. The frantic dash to the bathroom, the slamming of the door, the lifting of the toilet seat, the gagging, the retching, the splashing. The relief. The vows never to do this again. The breaking of those vows within hours.

I reveled in self-hatred and perfectionism. I refused to tuck in my shirt because I thought my stomach was too huge. I spent hours with my head craned around to better examine the expanse of my butt in the bathroom mirror. If I received a perfect score on an exam, it still wasn't good enough. I starved myself as punishment. I would speed in traffic because I was afraid the person behind me wouldn't like me if I wasn't driving fast enough. I spent hours studying and recopying my notes so they would have no mistakes and the handwriting would look "perfect." If I didn't know the answer to a question in class, I berated myself for hours, thinking I was stupid and incompetent. Even if I deemed one of my accomplishments "acceptable," I still lived in fear that the next time, I would certainly fail.

Eating disorders, then, are really not about food. They are about how you feel about yourself; they are about low self-esteem, a tremendous need to feel in control of yourself and your surroundings, unrelenting perfectionism, and an alienation of the mind from the body. They are also about a brain gone awry, frayed wires sparking and igniting as the brain is unable to process messages about food and anxiety normally. While an eating disorder usually begins as a deliberate act by the sufferer to lose weight in order to feel better, the eating disorder soon takes control of everything. As a person's problems become worse, the deeper one falls into the eating disorder. It's like living on a sinking ship, continually bailing out water, refusing to leave even as help arrives and the water level continues to rise. You still think you can save your leaky boat—you do not trust the help, you cannot see the shore that beckons, and you fear the life raft that is being thrown to you won't keep you from drowning. I can't guarantee that you will make it to shore if you abandon your leaky boat. But I can guarantee that you will surely drown if you do not let go.

Grabbing Hold of Recovery

All too often, I did not particularly want to recover. To someone without an eating disorder, this concept is baffling. How could you want to starve yourself to death? Yet, in my mind, food was like poison and gaining weight was tantamount to torture. If I ate, I would be *ordinary*. The hardest aspect of my recovery was the void

If I ate, I would be ordinary.

that was left behind as I let go of my eating disorder. Without anorexia, I was no one. Recovery was, in part, about creating an identity separate from the eating disorder with which I had shared a mind and body for so many years. (I did not let go of anorexia all at once, to be sure. Frequently, as life became more rocky, I'd fly right back into Ed's waiting arms.) But slowly, day by day, meal by meal, I gained confidence both in myself and in the skills that I was learning in treatment. Some days, staying in recovery involved making a phone call to my therapist or my mother or a friend. Other days, choosing recovery was as simple as picking up that fork and putting food in my mouth. Simple, yes. Easy? Never.

Initially, I had no choice but to recover. I was told "eat or die." Since it was made clear to me that my parents were not willing to stand around and watch me die, I began to eat. Then I began to hunger: for food, for *life*. I am still hungry for this. At times, I am overwhelmed by my hunger for things like friendship or even just a good cup of coffee.

Along with my eating disorder, I was forced to grapple with the true implications of two other psychiatric illnesses with which I had been diagnosed: bipolar disorder and obsessive-compulsive disorder (OCD). Anorexia had placed a buffer between the bipolar disorder and OCD and myself, as well as a buffer between myself and the rest of the world. When that buffer was wrenched away in treatment, everything within me was so raw that I felt my insides had been abraded with sandpaper. The world was very large and very unsafe and I was deeply fearful of what it would surely do to me. My obsessions and compulsions exploded. If I didn't drive around the block *just one more time*, then I could never be sure I hadn't hit someone with my car and left him or her to die by the side of the road. If I didn't arrange all of my belongings on my desk before bed each night, then something horrible would happen (I never could articulate what, precisely, that bad thing was). I despaired of anything good happening to me, ever. I thought about ending my own life many times.

I also had to endure the physical ramifications of years of starvation. I am 26, but have the bones of a 60-year-old woman. The osteoporosis is so severe that I have already broken three bones and had major ankle surgery. I developed epilepsy, and consequently lost my drivers license for a year and a half before my seizures were brought under control. My intestines stop working at the slightest provocation, worn down after long-term, heavy laxative abuse. Many times, I doubted recovery was worth it. All of the above happened after I was out of the grips of severe anorexia and bulimia; if this was recovery, why bother?

What brought me through? A combination of willingness and perseverance. I might not always have wanted to eat or gain weight (in fact, I can't think of a time in the early days when I did), but I was willing to give it a shot. I placed my trust in my treatment team and those who loved me. I white-knuckled it through more days than I care to count. I wanted to eat everything in sight; I never wanted to eat again. If I gained one pound, then I would gain a

I wanted to eat everything in sight; I never wanted to eat again.

hundred. Slowly, as I dimly realized that my appetite did not overwhelm me and that I could gain weight in a slow, controlled fashion, I began to relax. Just a little. Just enough to figure out what had motivated me to stop eating in the first place.

For me, the eating disorder brought with it a sense of accomplishment, a sense of safety and security, and a tempering of the waves of anxiety that so frequently washed over me. At least I could take action against my anxieties about food. I hoped that once I lost enough weight, I would finally feel "good enough." When I never did, I assumed it was simply because I was eating too much and hadn't lost enough weight. Then, when a small rational section of my mind realized that I had lost a life-threatening amount of weight, I just told myself how much better I would feel when I lost more.

The Face in the Mirror
My turning point came the day I looked in the mirror and saw what everyone else did: gaunt cheeks, sunken eyes, lips blue from the cold, and a thin layer of fur called *lanugo* covering me

from my eyebrows to my bellybutton. I realized I was staring into the face of death. I was staring into the face of an anorexic. I could no longer deny to myself that I had a problem. Actually taking a stand and doing something about the problem took another several years. In the interim, I was hospitalized twice and spent several months in residential care at a treatment facility in Philadelphia. I did better while in treatment, but promptly fell on my face the moment I was discharged (sometimes, within hours).

What compelled me to do this, you might ask? In some sense, there is no good answer. I didn't know how to approach life outside the narrow confines of anorexia and bulimia. I didn't know how to phone a friend and say "I'm having trouble." I didn't know how to value myself and my experiences. But what I slowly learned was that I could pick myself up each time I fell. I learned that "I can't" usually means "I won't," and that "I won't" usually means "I'm scared to." I became willing to chip away at the rock that was my eating disorder.

Slowly, over several long years, I did.

The rock is still there, to be sure. I still automatically scan menus at restaurants for salads and low-fat entrees; the difference is that I don't feel obligated to choose one of them. I still read labels on food packages; the difference is that I don't have rules about what I will and won't eat. I still watch cooking shows; the difference is that I don't sit in front of the TV for hours on end, drooling like a mindless zombie. I am also still anxious, extreme, and a perfectionist. I understand now that these are aspects of my personality that are inborn; they contributed to the eating disorder but, with practice, they can also be transformed into positive traits.

I have done much now that I am leaving my eating disorder behind. I published a memoir detailing my journey into and out of anorexia. I recently graduated with a master's degree in public health and infectious disease (an amusing choice for someone with hand-washing OCD), and plan to return to school to pursue a degree in science writing. I have a job, a cat, an apartment. Moreover, I have a life. I have reasons to get out of bed in the morning other than seeing what the scale reads. I have finally come to look in the mirror and like the person I see staring back at me. This person is not perfect, not by any stretch of the imagination, but she is me. Not "Carrie the Weight-Loss Wonder Goddess," nor a hopeless, chronic, incurable anorexic and bulimic. Just me.

Chapter Two

Evolution of an Eating Disorder

Even after years of therapy, I still can not describe how my eating disorder began and how it evolved the way it did. In a period of six months, I went from being a healthy college student to the brink of death from self-starvation. I do not know what sent me over the edge at that particular moment in time. Could it be that I was stressed out to the max, and suffering from a nasty bout of depression? That my OCD was once again flaring up? Perhaps. And perhaps it was a little more complicated than that.

What I can say is that my eating disorder was not caused by my parents (whom I love dearly), reading too many issues of fashion magazines (I don't even remember reading any), being sexually assaulted (though I was, at the age of 11), or being called "fatty" by other kids (that was also true, even though I was never remotely overweight). Were some of these contributing factors? Certainly. I cannot deny that. But I never set out to lose weight to win a man, to develop a certain "look," or to look like a model.

I thought that losing five pounds would just make me happy . . .

I thought that losing five pounds would just make me happy, finally make me acceptable to myself and to everyone else.

I nearly lost all semblance of life as a result.

In the Beginning

In some ways I fulfill all of the stereotypes of a person with an eating disorder: compulsive, neurotic, a perfectionist, a super-achiever. In others, I remain an enigma: crafter of sentences, cloner of genes, phobic of pasta. I was born into a white middle-class family in the suburbs of Detroit—a family whose history was fraught with mood and anxiety disorders. That, more than anything else, set me up for my future with both anorexia and bulimia.

My childhood was relatively uneventful. A born perfectionist and dreamer, I read books . . . and books and books and books. I was always at the top of my class, though few people thought I was particularly smart since I rarely spoke up. I was a daredevil in some areas, but rather socially anxious. I was *very* particular about certain things. Instead of chronicling my young life in a diary, I practiced my handwriting for hours on end, writing letters over and over and over again until they were "perfect." I would clip my nails in this same manner, until they were so short they bled almost continuously. I also had to organize all of my books by size, from tallest to shortest. I threw fits when any of my systems were broken.

I was never a small child, always taller and hence heavier than my classmates. That, combined with my love of learning and predilection toward shyness, essentially painted a bull's-eye on my back for any approaching bullies. And there were plenty. Confused at what was going on and not knowing any way to stop it, I learned to endure and keep a low profile. I increasingly found much solace in books as I moved through elementary school. A voracious reader, I would polish off up to 13 books in a week.

All hell broke loose, however, when I hit puberty. No one told me that girls are supposed to gain around 40 to 50 pounds at this time, or that people gain height and weight in different orders. I went through puberty relatively early, and reached my adult height and weight by the age of 12. This clearly distinguished me from my more petite classmates, and one boy in my class took advantage of this. He spared no opportunity to torment me about my weight and size. One day, seizing an opportunity when the teacher was out of the room, he shoved me up against the cinderblock wall at the back of the classroom and rummaged through my body, pinching and groping at inappropriate places. He stepped away just as the teacher entered the room. Fearing retribution, I told no one. I began to hate my body for simply existing. Shortly thereafter, I entered a bout of borderline anorexia, which subsided just as bizarrely as it had begun.

It was during these same years that I first began to suffer from depression. The onset was so insidious that many years had passed before I first noticed it as a problem. Didn't everyone feel this way? Wasn't it normal to hate life? I also suffered dramatic mood swings that were attributed to adolescence, though they were, in reality, the first inklings of the bipolar illness with which I would later be diagnosed (I will discuss problems that commonly co-occur with eating disorders more at length in Chapter 3).

As if normal teenage angst was not enough, I began encountering tremendous, unrelenting, and irrational fears about the details of everyday life—the first symptoms of obsessive-compulsive disorder. I was convinced that I had contracted AIDS and if I didn't wash my hands when they had been "contaminated," I would surely kill someone with my carelessness. I had to wash for exactly 55 seconds each time, restarting my ritual if I was interrupted. Soon, my hand washing had escalated to over 30 times per day, often with bleach or an abrasive cleaner. Any spare time I had was spent ruminating about what a horrible person I was, and how the only way to remedy this was to wash. I developed two rather conflicting fears: that I really did have AIDS and was destined to die a horrific, slow death; and that I was completely and utterly insane. Faced with this, I kept my washing a secret from everyone around me, including my parents. I often contemplated suicide, desperate for a way out of this hell.

I did gain control of my washing, only to have my obsessive-compulsive fears morph into different monsters: copying my school notes over and over and over, or repeatedly checking that I had turned off the coffee pot when I left the house. These fears waxed and waned over the years, and I never knew that my suffering wasn't normal or that its name was obsessive-compulsive disorder. I simply thought this was the way my life was destined to be. Though my OCD was debilitating, it also allowed me to flourish in school. I graduated high school as valedictorian and headed off to a small liberal arts school as a prospective biochemistry major.

I moved through college with the same frenetic speed I had gathered through high school. I had earned enough advanced placement credits to begin college as a sophomore, and took on a hefty 18 credits during my first semester. I also worked in a microbiology lab and as a part-time features editor at the college newspaper. These extracurricular activities proved to be rather effective distractions from my pervading sense of depression, anxiety, and self-loathing by providing a series of tasks that I felt I could accomplish relatively well. And accomplish them I did. To help deal with the stress of all of the continual work (and the boredom of typing at a computer for eight hours a day), I began to exercise regularly. It soon became a compulsion, though I never connected my increased activity with weight loss.

I spent the fall semester of my junior year studying health sciences at the University of Aberdeen in Scotland. It was as if someone had magically erased my whiteboard of anxiety and depression. To this day, I cannot explain this phenomenon. It gave me the opportunity to experience the best six months of my life. I learned how to play the bodhran (the Irish drum) from a slightly intoxicated Danish man in a pub; I fell hideously and hopelessly in love; I trespassed on sheep fields; I scaled waterfalls and stared into the churning Irish Sea for an hour. All of my carousing did, however, cause a slight weight gain. Not much, no more than five pounds. It was just barely enough to make my jeans a little tight around the waist. I returned to college determined to do something about that, to alleviate the anxiety caused by a pair of pants. So, at the remarkable age of 20, I decided rather innocently to lose five pounds. I have never regretted any action in my life as much as that one.

Just Five Pounds . . .

My eating disorder started out rather slowly, with the determination to exercise *every single day, dammit!*, and the inexorable exclusion of more and more foods from my diet. Items containing fat were the first to go, then meat, then pretty much anything with calories. Yet the changes were so gradual that I scarcely noticed until I was so

. . . the changes were so gradual that I scarcely noticed until I was so deep in anorexia that I couldn't extricate myself.

deep in anorexia that I couldn't extricate myself. In almost no time at all, I became downright phobic of food, and would only eat a small variety of foods I deemed "acceptable." In spite of my escalating eating disorder, I completed my spring semester having secured an internship that summer in the smallpox labs at the Centers for Disease Control and Prevention (CDC) in Atlanta, Georgia. I thought my life was finally falling into place: a fabulous internship, great chances to start a Ph.D. program in microbiology the following year, and weight loss on top of it all.

The only person who had any sense of foreboding of the months and years to come was my mother. She always asked if I was eating enough ("Yes, of *course* I am, Mom!"), and if I really wanted to go to Atlanta ("Why not?"). She reluctantly packed me off for the summer, having watched me grow thinner by the day. As I left home, the bottom dropped out of my life. I was seized and taken hostage by the eating disorder, and I had no way of stopping it, even if I'd wanted to.

Atlanta, GA

Life in Atlanta does not come back to me in a smooth, linear chronology. The memories arrive in brief spurts: a moment here, a recollection there, with whole days and weeks in between obliterated by anorexia. My existence in Atlanta was defined by my eating disorder. I remember, very clearly, the first time I flung my steering wheel to the right to go into the corner drugstore to buy laxatives; how my face burned crimson, and how I thought that if I read the directions on the box, I would somehow "protect" myself from any unwanted side effects. Five years later, I was still addicted to laxatives. I also remember what I ate every day. It never varied. As my life so quickly and inevitably fell down around me, the certainty of the calories I ate versus the calories I burned became the rock upon which my life was built.

The irony of my memories is how little I remember of my internship at the CDC, where I held a prestigious position working in the smallpox virus labs conducting classified government research (as in, "I'd tell you, but then I'd have to kill you"). I tested new vaccines and worked on bioterrorism research and new ways to identify strains of smallpox virus in the event that it was released. I do remember how much I truly enjoyed the work; it was interesting, and no one, anywhere else in the world, was doing what I did. The experiments have since been declassified, so, no, men in black suits and sunglasses are not going to be coming after me for writing this.

Simultaneously, both the depression and OCD worsened. Besides my obsessions and compulsions with food, I became a complete neat freak. I vacuumed my shared apartment several times a day, and then scoured out the sinks and the bathtub. Finally, before going to bed, I checked the front door lock five times, *precisely five times*. Four just wasn't good enough. I think my roommate thought I was a little cracked, but she had a large enough heart to like me anyway.

I broke down and saw a therapist because the anxiety that accompanied the anorexia-induced starvation was becoming unbearable, as was the loneliness of living in a strange city. I never had any intention of eating more, and certainly not of gaining weight. If anything, I wanted the anxiety and depression out of the way so I could shed a couple more pounds. So I did a little search on the Internet through an eating disorders treatment finder Web site and found a psychologist and called her up. I had never really been in therapy before, except for a brief stint at my college counseling center, so I had no idea how it worked or what one did to find a proper therapist. I lucked out. My therapist was awesome. We got along really well. It was hard for me to trust her at first, but she reminded me that this was normal, as she was a complete stranger—regardless of her credentials, experience, and degrees.

After a couple of sessions, she noticed my plummeting weight and deepening depression and suggested I consider more intensive treatment at a hospital. First, I had to get a medical workup and see a nutrition specialist. The session with the nutritionist was a joke. She told me how much someone of my age and activity level should be eating, which scared the living snot out of me. She then weighed me with my back to the scale (a common practice with eating disorder patients, to get the focus off how much you weigh), and told me how much weight I had to gain. After I got done freaking out in the parking lot, I drove home, crumpled up the menu she had given me, and threw it in the trash. I went to an urgent care clinic to have some blood work done, as well as an evaluation of my heart, since cardiac irregularities are common in persons with all types of eating disorders, particularly those who purge. They told me that a 20-year-old was too old to have anorexia, and that I couldn't be anorexic anyway since I wasn't wearing enough clothes (it was a humid 95 degrees outside, and I was shivering in jeans and a t-shirt). They handed back my irregular EKG and told me I just had a thyroid problem. I stomped out the door with my blood work results the next day.

They told me that a 20-year-old was too old to have anorexia, and that I couldn't be anorexic anyway since I wasn't wearing enough clothes ...

My therapist took one look at my lab results and requested I be hospitalized based on medical and psychological instability. I had very low blood pressure and a very low pulse because my body was so starved. I was also severely depressed and anxious and unable to begin eating on my own. I shrieked in protest: I had a job! I had school! I was turning 21 in less than a week! Screw this! I was *not* going to get fat!

My therapist looked at me and said quietly: You have a *life*.

I gulped. I stared at something interesting on the toe of my tennis shoe for about five minutes, turning this thought over and over in my head. I listened to the weak, irregular *thump* of my heart beneath my sternum.

I agreed to go into the hospital that next weekend.

Impatient Inpatient

Inpatient hospitalization can be beneficial, and indeed, all four times I was hospitalized, it saved my life. However, a hospital ward or treatment center is not camp. The first place I went was a psych ward. What I remember most was pulling my suitcase behind me, the nurse's hand gently on my elbow, and the door loudly clicking shut behind me. No way out. I was stuck. I was nuts. I was *one of Them*. The Crazy People. The people talked about at cocktail parties in hushed whispers punctuated with the occasional giggle.

This is one thing we forget, with all of the glamorization of eating disorders in the popular press: Eating disorders are serious psychiatric illnesses, and they are much more complex than a simple desire to be thin. I don't know anyone who deliberately tried to wind up hospitalized, or on an IV, or with tubes up their nose. If they did, there was already an underlying problem. Hospitals are not fun. Your bathroom will be locked. You will have to ask to pee. You will be monitored 24 hours a day, 7 days a week. Your food will be given to you on plastic trays and you will have to eat it. All of it. Even if you think it might taste like dog doo. (You will frequently be right about this.)

Hospitals can also be places of tremendous healing. You will be around people, maybe for the first time, who really get it. You will tell them secrets you have kept locked in your heart for a lifetime. You will yell, scream, cry, bitch, swear. You will challenge each other, you will trust, you will betray, you will be betrayed. It is like life, only on a smaller scale, with people who are much more intense and volatile.

It came as a great shock to my parents when I was released from my first hospitalization that I was not "fixed" or "cured." I was just as sick as when I went in. I did not want to get better, and so I didn't. Attitude is a big factor; so is supportive (and watchful) staff. I wanted to play games; I did, and I got away with it. My parents didn't find out about this until much later, and they were very pissy when they did. First at me, then at the hospital. However, I maintained the guise of health long enough to talk my way into going back to school, the point of which was, in my mind, simply to lose more weight.

Which I did. My weight at discharge was still dangerously low, and it didn't take much to push me over the edge. At this point, my intentions had long since surpassed any cute little euphemisms of "going on a diet" or "trying to lose a little weight." I was throwing out the baby with the bath water. I wanted to push my body to its ultimate limit, and the only way to find that limit was to go a little bit too far, to topple over the edge of the cliff and go into utter freefall.

I wanted to push my body to its ultimate limit, and the only way to find that limit was to go a little bit too far . . .

My memories of the few weeks I remained at college are even sketchier than when I lived in Atlanta. I have notes from my classes that I don't remember taking, homework I don't remember turning in, let alone completing. What I remember is this: My apartment was above a furniture store, a climb of five flights of stairs each time I wanted to come home. There was an elevator that I never used, fearing that someone would think me lazy if I used it. Then the cold—even as the August humidity melted into a sultry September, my very bones felt frigid. My nails and hands had a perpetual blue tinge that only disappeared on my daily runs and in my steaming hot showers. Lastly, there were the rumors. I had lost a sickening amount of weight over the summer, and one of the favorite topics of conversation as the fall semester started up on my small campus was what I was dying of. The top two votes were cancer and AIDS. No one guessed anorexia.

I was required to see a campus counselor as a condition of my return to college, which I dutifully did. I rolled my eyes about the whole thing. I told her how hard I was trying, eyeing her with my huge, green, puppy dog eyes. I don't know whether she bought a word I said. But several sessions later she told me that she wanted me to take a medical leave and seek inpatient treatment. Again. I goggled at her. Me? A college dropout?

"Carrie, we're talking about your *life* here."

I wondered, vaguely, if anyone had considered whether or not I wanted to live at that point.

I curled up in her overstuffed chair, shivering. She wrapped her jacket around me. I thought about how, earlier that day, I had stared at the face of death in the mirror. My own face. I had grown fur, my lips were now blue, I could see my dark sunken eyes and protruding cheekbones. I was blacking out regularly. I felt a horrible necrosis growing inside me. I was dying. And school didn't matter anymore.

I nodded. And filled out the forms. And moved out of my apartment.

It was September 2001. I spent most of my time laying about the house, occasionally licking at a light yogurt or nibbling an apple. I had given up, simply stopped caring. My mom began to look into treatment centers. Then, one bright sunny Tuesday morning, passenger planes turned into weapons and crashed into buildings and the entire world changed. I refused to get on a plane after that, and so my decision was made for me: I would check into a Philadelphia treatment center, a facility within driving distance of my parents' house.

Treatment in Philadelphia

Something in me shifted as I entered treatment for the second time. I had reached rock bottom (though the problem with rock bottom is, as writer Lolly Winston says, "There's always another layer of bargain basement junk"), and I knew it was eat or die. So I picked up the fork and began to eat. I felt some sort of minimal life force return. As I began to re-feed, my appetite returned with a vengeance. It frightened me. My metabolism surged so high, I would wake up in the middle of the night with hunger pains, drenched in sweat because I was burning calories at such a ferocious rate. I learned more about the origins of my eating disorder while in treatment, though I learned precious little about how to cope with it in the outside world. And when the two collided (treatment and the rest of reality), I flipped.

I had made progress up until that point, perhaps so much that my therapist thought I was far better off than I really was. I trusted neither her nor myself, so I didn't have an outlet for my intense, conflicting emotions. I coped by beginning to cheat on my meal plan. I had gained enough independence in the five weeks I had been at the treatment center that I had almost complete control over monitoring whether I had fulfilled my meal plan (or not) for the day. I started off small, saying I had two creamers in my coffee when I only had one. Then I grew more brazen and, simultaneously, more desperate. I began living on chef's salads and cottage cheese. And no one noticed. My weight gain slowed, and then stopped entirely. The more food the treatment facility told me I had to eat, the more I began to lie. I had dug myself into a hole from which I couldn't escape.

The more food the treatment facility told me I had to eat, the more I began to lie.

I had gained some much-needed weight during my two months in Philadelphia, but what I didn't get were coping skills that I could transfer to the outside world. So the glimmer of hope I had felt at the beginning of treatment dimmed and went black.

I didn't leave treatment determined to lose weight, just determined not to gain a single ounce. My problem was that I didn't have a scale, my dad having confiscated ours after I returned home from my first hospitalization. The only way I could be *absolutely sure* I wasn't gaining was to lose. Just a little. At least at first. I had set up a good, competent treatment team to see me upon my release from the center, but even they couldn't break through my anorexic mentality. I tried to work on my food fears, but my OCD anxieties and rituals kept interfering, and I lacked any meaningful strategies to conquer them. My therapist, though a wonderful woman with whom I did a lot of great work, focused more on my past than my present and future. I remained unsure of healthy ways to deal with my depression and anxiety in the here and now. I got a part-time job at the mall to give me something to do, and,

I figured, to give me more chances to skip meals and lose weight. It worked.

Hospitalization, Take Two

I was admitted to the psychiatric ward of a local hospital just after Christmas, my weight again dangerously low and continuing on a downward plunge. I stayed for two weeks, again experiencing the side effects of re-feeding. My stomach had shrunken so horribly that even normal-sized portions caused me cramping pains. I tried simply pushing the food around on my plate until I was told that I had to sit at the table until I had finished all of my food. I brought a book to read while my food cooled in front of me. It was neatly plucked out of my hands. I hurled insults at the nurse on duty. He raised his eyebrows in vague amusement, pulled up a chair, crossed his legs, and just waited. I stared at him, slack-jawed. Surely they were kidding.

Nope.

I finished my dinner. It was truly disgusting—fish nuggets, tater tots, and canned peas. This was not a meal to make one think that food is something to be enjoyed.

I returned to my room later, staring out the ninth floor window, looking at the busy Detroit streets and the headlights whizzing by, realizing no one gave a rip about an angry anorexic and mean doctors and nasty fish nuggets. It occurred to me that the world did not revolve around my dinner plate. I had received a letter from my college roommate, asking me if I could please come back to her because she missed me when I was so deep into the anorexia. I sat on my bed and thought about all this. I realized that my roommate was using million-dollar pieces of equipment in chemistry lab, while I was not even trusted with safety scissors. I couldn't even feed myself. I realized, in that moment, how utterly pathetic my existence had become.

I became determined to beat my eating disorder.

What I didn't know was how much more work I had in front of me, and that wishes don't necessarily make dreams come true.

Chapter Three

The Basics: What You Need to Know About Eating Disorders

What is an eating disorder, and where does it come from? Is it simply a bunch of food or diet junkies waiting to get their next fix? Is it young men and women who have been seduced by magazine images and want to look like Barbie and Ken? Is it a brain disease? Could it all be in our heads? Could we be doing it "just for attention"?

Well, yes. And no.

No one knows for sure the exact origins of eating disorders, and it's very likely that there isn't one single cause. Much of the current scientific literature on eating disorders suggests that psychological factors such as low self-esteem, a genetic predisposition toward mental illness (especially anxiety disorders), and a society that encourages dieting and thinness may all collide to cause eating disorders in some men and women. One thing is for sure, though: Eating disorders are among the most dangerous of psychiatric disorders and may claim more lives each year than any other mental illness.

Eating Disorders Defined

The two most talked-about eating disorders are anorexia and bulimia. Also affecting young people is binge eating disorder (uncontrollably eating large amounts of food in a short period of time). While these disorders have specific criteria used by mental health professionals and insurance companies, many people with a diagnosable eating disorder fall into the category of eating disorder not otherwise specified (EDNOS). People with EDNOS can still have serious and life-threatening eating problems, even though they might not be classified strictly as "anorexic" or "bulimic."

Anorexia Nervosa

It is believed that anorexia occurs in approximately 1% of women at some point in their lives. While the numbers are less certain in adolescents, a recent study estimated that about 0.5% of teenage American girls have anorexia nervosa. Prevalence rates in men and boys are about one-tenth of those observed in women. People suffering from anorexia are unable to consume enough calories to maintain a normal, healthy body weight. They may restrict their food to only a fraction of the amount they need to keep body and mind working normally. Another common aspect of anorexia is excessive and/or compulsive exercise, where an individual's entire life is ruled by how much time she spends exercising in order to burn calories. Some people with anorexia also engage in binge eating and purging behaviors, such as self-induced vomiting or laxative and diuretic abuse. The latest edition of the *Diagnostic and Statistical Manual of Mental Disorders*, Fourth Edition (*DSM-IV,* the diagnostic bible of the mental health world), has identified two different subtypes of anorexia: anorexia nervosa restricting (AN-R), for when sufferers maintain a low weight mainly through caloric restriction and excessive exercise, and anorexia nervosa binge eating/purging (AN-BP), for those who also engage in binge eating and/or purging.

As starvation sets in and continues, people with anorexia can become frenetic with determination to lose more and more weight. Sometimes, sufferers will constantly exercise or move as an attempt to burn more calories. Even as I watched the numbers drop on the scale and dropped clothing sizes, I couldn't see the difference in the mirror. Every day, I followed a rigid exercise routine and had great anxiety when I missed a workout. I almost couldn't sit still. My psychiatrist once told me that laboratory rats deprived of food in experiments became hyperactive, presumably on a search to find food. Sufferers can use layers of baggy clothing to disguise weight loss (or, in my case, baggy clothes were from lack of money to buy a new wardrobe). It is also an attempt to stay warm as the metabolism slows down to preserve energy. My body also began to grow fine, downy lanugo to help conserve precious heat.

Many different personality changes can accompany anorexia. My obsessions and compulsions multiplied, and I began measuring all of my food, counting calories, fat grams, fiber, and sodium, using a little notebook to keep track of everything that I ate. I ate the same few foods in the same order at the same time each day. I also

Many different personality changes can accompany anorexia.

developed OCD behaviors that were completely unrelated to food and weight, like scouring every surface in the apartment every single day. I grew deeply depressed, withdrawing from friends and family, crying myself to sleep every night because I could not see a way out of this misery. I got irritated easily and snapped at random people. But the promise of a lower number on the scale in the morning drew me further and further into anorexia.

Many of the side effects of anorexia are psychological because, gram for gram, the brain consumes the most energy of any organ in the body. Even as it became obvious that I was starving and emaciated, I failed to believe there was a problem. Not eating wasn't the problem, it was the solution. I did exactly what I set out to do: lose weight. A lot of it. And I certainly had no intention of stopping. Only when my family stepped in and refused to let me starve myself to death did it begin to sink in that I was seriously ill.

Recent studies have shown that anorexia has a strong association with certain personality traits like neuroticism, and other mental illnesses such as obsessive-compulsive disorder. Many of the symptoms of anorexia, such as obsessionality, depression, and anxiety, have been noted in otherwise healthy individuals who are on very low calorie diets, causing the "chicken and the egg" dilemma: Are people suffering from anorexia just exacerbating their innate personality traits? Or does the disease itself create them?

Bulimia Nervosa

Bulimia nervosa is thought to affect around 1% to 5% of teenage American girls, while up to 3% of women will be bulimic at some point in their lives. Again, the numbers for men are about a tenth of those observed in women. People suffering from bulimia engage in a cycle of binge eating followed by purging to get rid of the food, and to relieve the subsequent guilt and anxiety. Purging can involve self-induced vomiting, laxative and diuretic abuse, and extreme fasting and compulsive exercise. Many times, the sufferer will use more than one method to "undo" the binge. This cycle rapidly becomes addictive and impossible to control. The cycle of binge eating and purging can become all-consuming, with the majority of waking hours spent planning the next binge and figuring out how and where to purge.

In my own episodes of binge eating, I found a certain amount of relief from the depression and anxiety I was experiencing. The purging that followed the binge then relieved the anxiety and guilt I felt after having consumed such a large number of calories, as well as relieving the physical discomfort of the binge.

As I slid into bulimia during my pseudo-recovery from anorexia, the binge eating and purging soon spiraled out of control. All I could think of was my next binge and my next purge. It demarcated my day: the order of food I would eat as I binged, the post-binge bathroom ritual. I was deeply ashamed of my behaviors and my desperate need for vast volumes of sweets. I vowed to stop almost every single day. Most of the time, my efforts were in vain. It was only when I confessed my binge eating and purging rituals to my dietician that anyone found out that I had developed bulimia.

Partly in order to ensure I wouldn't binge, and partly to make up for the previous day's binge eating and purging, I greatly restricted my food intake. However, this creates a physiological deprivation of energy and nutrients and consequently drives the urge to binge. "The best way to head off a binge," my dietician tells me, "is simply to eat." In persons whose diets are low in carbohydrates, binges may consist of sweets and other foods with simple sugars. When I wasn't consuming enough fat in my normal diet, I binged on foods with a high fat content. I wasn't crazy, and neither is anyone

"The best way to head off a binge," my dietician tells me, "is simply to eat."

with bulimia. We're responding, in part, to our body's desire for particular nutrients.

However, the continual fluctuation in brain chemicals from both binge eating and purging can cause rapid changes in moods. I was bright and sunny one minute, and depressed and sobbing the next. My purging caused sudden and unexpected dehydration and a loss of potassium (vomiting, laxatives, and diuretics can all cause both these problems). I grew frantic and anxious if I couldn't purge after a binge. I was hysterical, sobbing and crying, but afraid to tell anyone why.

Though not useful for anorexia, various medications have proved useful for bulimia, helping to decrease the frequency of binges and purges; the only medication officially approved by the FDA to treat bulimia nervosa is Prozac (fluoxetine). I'll discuss medications for eating disorders more in Chapter 4.

EDNOS

Eating disorder not otherwise specified has been called a "grab bag" for all of the other eating disorders that don't neatly fit within the strict definitions of anorexia or bulimia. This has nothing to do with the seriousness of the eating disorder. There are as many hospital admissions for EDNOS as there are for anorexia or bulimia, and you can still die from this condition. Though I have suffered from both anorexia and bulimia, I was diagnosed with EDNOS when I was the sickest and nearly died. It's easy to think of EDNOS as not a real eating disorder (I'm guilty as charged), but the psychological and medical complications are just as serious.

Some people with EDNOS have all the most common characteristics of anorexia or bulimia, but do not meet one or two of the criteria required for an official diagnosis of that disorder. Others have more mixed features, such as being of normal weight but purging without binge eating, or repeatedly chewing and spitting out (without swallowing) large amounts of food.

Binge eating disorder, which involves binge eating followed not by purging but instead by immense guilt and even shame, also falls under the category of EDNOS. Though it is not recognized formally as its own separate illness in the *DSM-IV*, there has been increasing interest in binge eating disorder on the part of researchers, especially in connection with rising obesity rates and other major health complications. A recent report by the National Institute of Diabetes and Digestive and Kidney Diseases estimated that as many as four million Americans have binge eating disorder; it also stated that women are slightly more likely than men to be binge eaters.

For much of the time I was suffering from my eating disorder, my diagnosis was EDNOS. I would restrict a little, binge a little, overexercise a little, and purge a little—a strange amalgamation of symptoms that were both physically and mentally destructive. From the outside, I was a highly functioning, normal-looking young woman. I didn't "look" like I had an eating disorder . . . yet I very much did. Someone with an eating disorder can be a normal weight, which allows the illness to lurk for many, many years. However, persons suffering from EDNOS are just as in need of intensive help as are those suffering from anorexia and bulimia.

What Causes Eating Disorders?

The plain fact is that no one knows for sure what causes eating disorders. It appears that many different factors interact to cause them. I have been told that my eating disorder was caused by "family dysfunction," although my family is pretty functional. I have been told that the eating disordered thoughts were from Satan and I needed to repent or I was going to hell (to which I said, "Lady, I'm already in hell. Threats of going there really fail to frighten me"). Some people blame the media, and though the "never too thin" culture is certainly a factor, it doesn't explain why some people develop eating disorders and others don't; nor does it explain the fact that anorexia nervosa was first recognized and named in 1874—long before the advent of fashion magazines and supermodels.

Traditionally, eating disorders have been thought of as the upper-middle-class, white, teenaged girl's disease; she is also typically blonde, good-looking, and a cheerleader. While I am middle class, and developed the first signs of my eating disorder in my teens, I am not blonde, nor was I a cheerleader. I am a self-described geek. The simple fact is that eating disorders do not discriminate. A person of any age, race, ethnicity, gender, or socioeconomic class can develop an eating disorder.

If eating disorders were caused by one particular factor, then it would appear in *all* persons with eating disorders. However, that does not appear to be the case. What tends to occur are multiple influences, called "risk factors," that come together to cause anorexia and/or bulimia. There have been recent studies that identified both brain and biochemical causes as well as certain personality traits as potential culprits in causing an eating disorder. Other characteristics, such as gender, culture, and psychological factors, can add to this mixture and influence the chances of developing an eating disorder. One researcher says that "genes load the gun, and an environment pulls the trigger" when it comes to eating disorders. I like to think of eating disorders as a type of recipe: If you add the right ingredients and bake them for the right time, you can pull an eating disorder out of the oven. I've found that my efforts toward recovery don't depend as much on how and why I developed anorexia and bulimia as on what steps I can take to break free from the disease.

But this information is important because it helps researchers understand these illnesses and develop ways to prevent them.

Just because there is no one single cause of eating disorders doesn't mean experts don't know what factors *do* increase the risk of developing one. A number of biological, social, and psychological risk factors have been identified in the development of eating disorders. While many possible risk factors have been identified, scientific research has only recently honed in on the major ones, described below.

Gender

While the majority of people with anorexia and bulimia are female, a number of males have eating disorders, too. Males account for about one in ten eating disorder diagnoses, and some researchers believe the number of boys and men with eating disorders is on the rise, partly attributed to increased awareness by professionals. Some of the difference in numbers is attributed to the sociocultural pressures on girls to be thin, though boys are now facing similar pressures to look a certain way. Biological differences have also been proposed, though they have neither been clarified nor proven. Another likely reason for this gender difference is the higher proportion of girls and women who are on weight-loss diets, a major risk factor in the development of an eating disorder, which is discussed below.

... some researchers believe the number of boys and men with eating disorders is on the rise ...

Puberty

The most common age of onset of an eating disorder is during puberty, a time of great hormonal and physical changes to the body. The physical changes during puberty, especially in girls, may conflict with societal ideals of thinness and the boy-like models on the covers of magazines. Hormones may also set off waves of other biological changes that can affect the beginnings of an eating disorder. In general, anorexia nervosa tends to begin at a younger age than bulimia nervosa, but there are always exceptions. Young children (ages 10 and below), as well as people 35 and over, are now being diagnosed with eating disorders.

Brain Chemistry

Recent studies have discovered marked differences in the brain circuitry of women with eating disorders and women without, especially in the use of serotonin, a chemical brain messenger (known as a neurotransmitter) very much involved with mood and anxiety regulation. However, studies have not been able to determine whether this difference existed before the onset of the eating disorder or as a result of eating disordered behavior. A new study of persons who have entirely recovered from anorexia nervosa has shown serotonin abnormalities, pointing toward the idea that dysfunctions in serotonin pre-dated the eating disorder and somehow increased the likelihood of developing anorexia. Similarities between both anorexia and bulimia and obsessive-compulsive disorder (which is also associated with abnormalities in serotonin) have been noted. A preexisting anxiety disorder is also a major risk factor in the development of anorexia nervosa.

Genetics

Much of the new research on eating disorders has been focusing on genetics, that is, the particular innate factors that make us who we are and are inherited from generation to generation. A *genetic predisposition* is an inborn risk of a certain disease or disorder. You didn't cause it. Your parents didn't cause it. Some people have a genetic predisposition toward diabetes, or toward diseases like depression, and the same goes for eating disorders. Relatives of people with anorexia and bulimia are significantly more likely to develop an eating disorder themselves than people whose relatives do not have these illnesses, so it is clear that eating disorders run in families. There is also a significantly increased likelihood of EDNOS in these families, which means the genetic basis for an eating disorder is fairly broad. As well, twin studies demonstrate that an eating disorder is much more likely to occur in *both* identical twins, who share the exact same DNA, than in fraternal twins, who have only half of their DNA in common. All of this combined provides good evidence that eating disorders tend to run in families.

Is everyone's eating disorder related to genetics? I can't answer that question, and neither can researchers at this time. No single gene has been identified as a cause for either anorexia or bulimia. It is likely that there are several genes involved in the onset of these eating disorders, some of which are related to eating and appetite, others of which are related to depression and anxiety, and still others that control different aspects of behavior. Twin studies have shown that eating disorders are 50% to 70% inherited, but this doesn't mean that 50% to 70% of eating disorders are caused by genetics alone. It means that at least half of the risk for developing an eating disorder is related to genetic and individual variations in brain chemicals, while the rest involves contributions from the environment.

Psychological Factors and Personality Traits

People with anorexia are stereotyped as rigid, obsessive, perfectionist, and people-pleasing. Those with bulimia tend to be portrayed as impulsive, more inwardly perfectionist, and novelty-seeking. While it remains unclear exactly what role certain psychological factors play in the development of an eating disorder, research has shown that there are certain personality traits and thinking styles that are found more frequently in people with eating disorders than in the general population.

Recent studies have shown that anxiety disorders, obsessionality, and low self-esteem are linked to the development of anorexia.

Recent studies have shown that anxiety disorders, obsessionality, and low self-esteem are linked to the development of anorexia. Self-esteem plays a key role—many young people with eating disorders report not feeling satisfied about who they are, even disliking or hating themselves. Especially in a thin-oriented society, losing weight seems an easy way to feel more positive about who you are. Also playing a role is perfectionism, which is a need to do things "perfectly." Studies show that people who have fully recovered from anorexia tend to be more perfectionistic and have more anxiety than people who have never had an eating disorder, leading researchers to believe that these personality traits likely predated the development of the eating disorder. The problem with perfectionism is that nothing is ever good enough, or perfect enough, and this can trap a person in a cycle of dissatisfaction and self-hatred. Extreme perfectionism is an example of all-or-nothing thinking, also known as black and white thinking. Something is "good" or it is "bad"—there is no in between. To use myself as an example, if I didn't get a perfect score on a test, I was a failure. When I got my first A- in college, I locked myself in my room and cried for a week.

Another psychological risk factor is obsessionality and anxiety. While all of us are obsessed with different things (a particular band, a color, even foods), obsessionality refers to when a person constantly thinks about particular fears or objects, such as germs or numbers, even when doing so is no longer pleasurable. As I will discuss later in this chapter, obsessionality is closely related to obsessive-compulsive disorder.

Unfortunately, as with other risk factors, there is no simple connection between psychology, personality traits, and eating disorders. Although researchers can identify certain specific personality traits that are associated with anorexia and bulimia, not every person with those traits will go on to develop an eating disorder. Rather, it is likely that the interaction of an individual's particular psychological makeup with many other factors combine to cause an eating disorder.

Sociocultural Factors: The "Thin Ideal" and the Role of the Media

Current Western societies encourage thinness as both a health and a moral issue. Most diet products are selling the idea that if you aren't thin, you can't be happy—that there is something wrong with you. Unfortunately, many people equate their worth with their weight. Typically, however, the fashion models that display this "ideal" thinness are *underweight*, and promote an unhealthy image for women and men. As a result, most women, and an increasing percentage of men, have dieted in the past or are currently on a diet because they seek to emulate these models.

Does a culture's emphasis on thinness increase a person's risk of developing an eating disorder? This is certainly a common assumption, relentlessly reinforced by the media, with the smiling, ultra-thin models on glossy cover pages and the stories on celebrities who lose drastic amounts of weight. Even though I don't read fashion magazines, I am not unaware of this idea.

I always knew (somehow) that thin was better than fat, and that only thin girls in my school were popular. I never felt I could truly be successful unless I was thin. The irony is, of course, that I was both—thin and successful. More athletic-looking than bone thin, I still had a very healthy weight for my height. According to images in magazines and on TV, however, I was "overweight." Many times, the desire to look a certain way or even just "lose five pounds" can trigger an eating disorder. One psychologist has repeatedly pointed out that "normal" dieting and exercise cause chemical changes in a person's brain that may make him or her more susceptible to developing an eating disorder.

While the diet mentality is dangerous enough, it wasn't strict weight loss that I was looking for when I decided to lose a few pounds. It was the mantra of "if you lose weight, you will be happy." I had seen the "before" and "after" pictures in the weight loss ads, and though I thought the idea vaguely ludicrous, I was so depressed that I was willing to try it. Some of the weight loss was unintentional, due to the depression I was experiencing at the time, but it made me feel better. I was *doing something*. That was not a cure-all for my depression, and as my nutrition decreased, the depression increased.

The fact that eating disorders are more common in Western societies suggests that the thin ideal is involved in the onset of eating disorders. However, people in almost every country have been found with diagnosable eating disorders, even in those countries without a strong emphasis on thinness. The rate of eating disorders in these countries is lower than that found in the United

... people in almost every country have been found with diagnosable eating disorders, even in those countries without a strong emphasis on thinness.

States or Europe, partially confirming the importance of an environment that encourages unhealthy weights for women and men. In the end, the thin ideal is important in the development of eating disorders, but it can't be the only factor driving their occurrence.

Race and Socioeconomic Status

Eating disorders, specifically anorexia nervosa, have been traditionally thought of as only affecting white upper-class females. However, the number of minorities diagnosed with eating disorders has been steadily increasing, and it is also apparent that an eating disorder does not look at your income before striking. Neither anorexia nor bulimia appears to discriminate in any way.

Dieting

Dieting is one of the most discussed—yet one of the least specifically defined—risk factors for an eating disorder. Part of the problem is that the word "diet" can mean many different things. While most uses of the word "diet" in our society refer to a specific effort to decrease food intake in an effort to lose weight, the medical use of the word "diet" means a person's overall eating habits. People can have different diets based on medical conditions, religious practices, and allergies. As my best friend from high school says, "A diet isn't something you're on; it's something you have."

As my best friend from high school says, "A diet isn't something you're on; it's something you have."

While this use of the word "diet" sounds ideal, it is the term *dieting* that is officially associated with deliberate and prolonged restriction of calories in order to lose weight. Many people with eating disorders report this type of behavior prior to the onset of the full-blown disorder. People can have a diet mindset without actually losing weight, by classifying certain foods as "good" or "bad", or avoiding certain foods. Dieting is extremely common in our society, especially among women. Polls have found that most women say they would like to lose weight or are unhappy with their current weight. One study in

Eating Disorder or Diet?

Dieting is about losing a little bit of weight in a healthy way.

Eating disorders are about trying to make your whole life better through food and eating (or lack of).

Dieting is about doing something healthy for yourself.

Eating disorders are about seeking approval and acceptance from everyone through negative attention.

Dieting is about losing a bit of weight and doing it healthfully.

Eating disorders are about how life won't be good until a bit (or a lot) of weight is lost, and there's no concern for what kind of damage you do to yourself to get there.

Dieting is about losing some weight in a healthy way so how you feel on the outside will match how good you already feel on the inside.

Eating disorders are about being convinced that your whole self-esteem is hinged on what you weigh and how you look.

Dieting is about attempting to control your weight a bit better.

Eating disorders are about attempting to control your life and emotions through food/lack of food—and are a huge neon sign saying "look how out of control I really feel."

Dieting is about losing some weight.

Eating disorders are about everything going on in life—stress, coping, pain, anger, acceptance, validation, confusion, fear—and cleverly (or not so cleverly) hidden behind phrases like "I'm just on a diet."

(Information courtesy of the Something Fishy Web site on eating disorders.)

2001 reported that 24% of girls and 17% of boys in the *third grade* claimed to be on a diet. Due to the seeming universality of dieting and the diet mindset, many eating disorders can be masked to parents and friends as "just another teenage diet."

Because the actual characteristics that determine whether or not a person is dieting are hard to define, it is unclear how much these are related to the development of an eating disorder. What has been identified as a risk factor for eating disorders is *unhealthy weight-loss behavior*—activities closely associated with a risk of physical harm, such as: self-induced vomiting; laxative, diuretic, and diet pill abuse; fasting; and excessive exercise to lose weight. Considering that a large number of teens and young adults engage in these behaviors, and that these behaviors can often lead to an eating disorder, it is likely that unhealthy weight-loss behaviors can signal the beginnings of a full-blown eating disorder.

Activities with a Focus on Body Shape and Weight

Sports such as ballet, wrestling, track, and gymnastics tend to be described as breeding grounds for eating disorders. While many people participate in these activities as part of a healthy lifestyle and do not develop eating disorders, such as I did for a number of years, dancers have been found to have diagnosable cases of anorexia nervosa that are 4 to 25 times higher than the general population. Other people, such as models, actresses, and entertainers, whose physical appearance is emphasized as part of their careers, are also more likely to develop an eating disorder. However, it may be hard to separate cause and effect. These fields could attract athletes and artists already suffering from a preoccupation with food and weight, or other risk factors that contributed both to their career choices and to the development of an eating disorder.

Family Relationships

In the 1950s, virtually all mental illnesses (including eating disorders) were assumed to be caused by particular patterns of family interactions early in a person's life. Although these theories were never confirmed in scientific research, many clinicians still place a high value on family interactions in both the origins and treatment of an eating disorder. By the time an eating disordered person shows up for treatment, there is often family dysfunction. Sometimes, it predates the eating disorder, other times it is magnified by the stresses of having an ill child. This isn't to say that a traumatic event in a family's life, such as death or divorce, will automatically trigger an eating disorder, or that all persons with eating disorders come from dysfunctional families. Some do, some don't. No family is perfect, and family therapy is useful in creating an environment that will best help you recover from your eating disorder.

Peer Influence

Most teens place a pretty high value on friends and social life, so it's no wonder that peer influence (or what is often referred to as *peer pressure*) might increase the risk of developing an eating disorder. If a person's friends have exhibited excessive concern over body image, weight, and dieting, it stands to reason that that person will be more likely to adopt the same attitudes. Experts call this phenomenon "contagion," though no formal studies have yet been conducted to prove that it plays a part in causing an eating disorder.

Childhood Trauma

Much attention has been given to the role of childhood trauma, particularly sexual abuse, in the development of an eating dis-

What's New in Eating Disorders Research

For many years, eating disorders were thought to be caused by over-controlling mothers, a society that told women "Be thin or else!," or a desire to remain a child, among other factors. While all of these issues can contribute to eating disorders in certain people, much of the current research on both anorexia and bulimia has focused on the biochemical and genetic influences on these diseases. Anorexia and bulimia have independently been linked to differences in the levels of serotonin and dopamine (neurotransmitters involved in feeling pleasure) in the brain. While some of these differences could be side effects of the disorders themselves, they also likely predate the eating disorder and may continue after a person has successfully recovered. Likewise, genetic influences have been implicated in the risk of developing an eating disorder, though it is likely that this effect is not limited to any single gene. Many studies are finding that, in any type of eating disorder, genetics plays a far larger role than was anticipated many years ago. Studies have also shown that the increasing emphasis on thinness and dieting may also be attributed to the development of an eating disorder. As well, many people diagnosed with an eating disorder, even those in their teens, have another co-occurring psychiatric diagnosis, such as depression, OCD, or substance abuse.

In addition to investigations into the causes and origins of eating disorders, cutting-edge research is also being done on new and more effective ways to diagnose, prevent, and treat these disorders. Here are some examples:

- *Work continues on tracking down the precise genetic traits that may increase a person's chances of developing an eating disorder.* A new study has identified six core traits (obsessionality, age at menarche, anxiety, lifetime body mass index [BMI], concern over mistakes, and food-related obsessions) that are associated with eating disorders, as well as genes that may be associated with these traits.
- *New, more reliable diagnostic tests are being developed,* including using hair analysis to detect anorexia and bulimia.
- *Research on new medications for treatment of eating disorders continues.* While antidepressants like Prozac have demonstrated an ability to decrease urges to binge and purge in people with bulimia, they have not shown any efficacy in helping

(*continued*)

those with anorexia either restore or maintain a healthy body weight. Studies on the use of atypical antipsychotics to decrease body image distortion as well as anorexic behaviors are ongoing. (Medications for eating disorders are discussed further in Chapter 4.)

- *A new way to help prevent bulimia in high-risk college students shows promise.* An online cognitive behavioral therapy program (cognitive behavioral therapy is discussed in more detail in Chapter 4) helped to decrease the number of high-risk college students who developed bulimia nervosa. This is the first such study that has shown any effect in truly preventing the onset of an eating disorder.

order. Recent studies have found that individuals with eating disorders are indeed more likely to have a history of traumatic experiences. However, not every person with an eating disorder has been through trauma, so a diagnosis of anorexia or bulimia does not mean that a person was sexually abused (or traumatized in other ways). It also doesn't mean that they weren't. Sadly, sexual abuse and other traumas are rather common among young women, and there is undoubtedly some crossover in these two populations. Although I was assaulted as a child, I still can't figure out the exact importance of this event on the development of my eating disorder. As well, the occurrence of childhood trauma increases a person's chances of developing a wide range of emotional and behavioral problems, so trauma can be viewed as a nonspecific risk factor for many problems that can occur later in life.

Medical Dangers

The medical complications of any eating disorder, no matter how long the duration and/or intensity, can be severe and, at times, fatal. The main dangers of eating disorders are caused by starvation (malnutrition) or result from unsafe behaviors like purging. There are also complications from binge eating disorder. Even young people who don't strictly fall into the diagnostic categories of eating disorders as defined by *DSM-IV* may still be at risk for developing some or all of these complications if they engage in unhealthy weight-control behaviors. Self-starvation is particularly damaging to young people who are still growing; adolescents may never reach their full height because of impeded bone development resulting from malnutrition.

As the body slows down due to lack of energy, many unhealthy physical changes take place. Both heart rate and blood pressure drop (known as bradycardia and hypotension) and the heart muscle is weakened. Purging also causes electrolyte imbalances that can cause sudden cardiac arrest. The size of the stomach shrinks and digestion slows as the intestines forget how to properly digest food. Constipation is also common. Menstruation may cease so that the body can conserve precious energy (this is called *amenorrhea*). Without necessary calcium and fat in the diet, bones can weaken and become brittle, causing osteoporosis even in teens and young adults. When glucose (the body's primary fuel) isn't available for use, the body begins to break down fats into small chemicals known as *ketones*. Ketones can be measured in the urine. They also cause bad breath, a concrete sign that the body is starving and not receiving enough energy. I personally have experienced all of these side effects.

Some other complications of self-starvation are:

- Low body temperature (plus blue finger and toenails, also lips)
- Fine, downy hair covering the body (especially the face and trunk)
- Easy bruising

- Fainting
- Fatigue and/or insomnia
- Iron deficiency (anemia)
- Decreased ability to fight infections
- Muscle atrophy
- Dehydration
- Seizures

Many of these complications, either on their own or in combination, can be fatal. Complications from purging can be equally serious:

- Dehydration (caused by vomiting, laxative, and/or diuretic abuse)
- Low levels of potassium and sodium
- Tears in the esophagus from vomiting
- Gastric rupture (fatal in 80% of cases)
- Calluses on the back of the hand from self-induced vomiting
- Cathartic colon (an inability to have normal bowel movements due to dependency on laxatives)
- Pancreatitis (an inflammation of the pancreas, which helps to regulate digestion)
- Edema (fluid retention)
- Kidney damage
- Seizures
- Erosion of tooth enamel from repeated vomiting
- Cardiac abnormalities

These dangers are not meant to be used as a "checklist" to determine how many of these you can rack up before considering yourself "sick enough." *Any* of these signs need to be checked out by a qualified physician with whom you can be honest about any and all of your eating disorder behaviors. Frequently, sufferers can be very ill and still have essentially normal laboratory results. This happened to me. However, electrolytes (such

> *Frequently, sufferers can be very ill and still have essentially normal laboratory results.*

as potassium and sodium) can fall to dangerous levels very quickly and cause sudden death. Normal blood work does not equal good health, nor does a "normal" weight.

Diseases That Frequently Co-occur with Eating Disorders

Many young people diagnosed with anorexia or bulimia are also found to have other mental disorders at the same time, myself included. Across all age groups, 70% of those with anorexia nervosa and 75% of those with bulimia nervosa are affected by other emotional, behavioral, and psychological problems. These problems, called *comorbidities* by health professionals, can predate the eating disorder, or develop after the eating disorder has begun. Whatever the case, these other conditions, which may have similar behaviors and thought patterns as the eating disorder, can take years to diagnose, and can complicate or delay the diagnosis and treatment of the eating disorder itself.

Such illnesses commonly include:

Mood Disorders

Significant mood disturbances such as major depressive disorder and bipolar disorder commonly co-occur with both anorexia and bulimia. Depression in particular tends to accompany eating disorders in many individuals. According to the *DSM-IV*, major depression essentially means that one is depressed or irritable nearly all the time, and/or has lost interest or enjoyment in almost everything. It's much worse than a simple case of the blues, and a person who is depressed can't just "snap out of it". It lasts for at least two weeks and is associated with other symptoms, such as a change in eating or sleeping habits, lack of energy, feelings of worthlessness, trouble with concentration, or thoughts of suicide. A diagnosis of major depression is not appropriate when an individual is depressed because of bereavement following the death of a loved one.

What to Do If You Are Feeling Suicidal

If you are feeling severely depressed and are having thoughts of ending your own life, you may feel that you do not deserve help, or even that you don't want it. You may feel all alone and that no one cares. However, there are still positive things you can do when you feel like you can't go on.

Call a friend or family member. My former roommate has been suicidal, and I've talked with her long into the night. I never once minded doing this. Put yourself in their shoes: If it were your friend, wouldn't you want to help?

Call your doctor or therapist. Most doctors and therapists allow their patients to call them anytime in an emergency. This is part of their job. If they don't answer, leave a message. If you really need to talk to someone, then:

- **Call a hotline.** It sounds cliché, but there really is always someone who cares. There are two 24-hour hotlines available that are staffed by volunteers trained to listen: The National Hopeline Network at 1-800-SUICIDE (784-2433) is a great toll-free resource that you can all from anywhere in America. There is also the National Suicide Prevention Lifeline, at 1-800-273-TALK (8255). A hotline can also connect you with a crisis center in your area.
- **Call 911.** Tell them you are feeling suicidal and don't think you can keep yourself safe. They will talk to you and help you decide on a course of action, including transport to the emergency room.

Bipolar disorder (also known as manic-depressive illness) alternates between periods of severe depression and periods of mania. Mania is characterized by an overly elevated or "high" mood, and other attributes such as inflated self-esteem, irritability, racing thoughts, a decreased need for sleep, and over-engaging in pleasurable and/or risky activities (such as excessive shopping, alcohol or drug abuse, and sex). Hypomania is similar to mania, only less intense and less disruptive. Episodes of mania and depression are a sign of bipolar I disorder, while hypomania and depression are signs of bipolar II disorder. The mood swings between depression and mania/hypomania can occur with no outside trigger, and are noticeable to friends, family, and co-workers.

I suffered from a severe depression, which was later diagnosed as bipolar II disorder due to episodes of hypomania, in which I had an extremely high mood, was very irritable, and felt less of a need for sleep and food. My eating disorder cycled in intensity with my moods, getting worse during depressive phases and improving during episodes of hypomania. My mood would always crash back down as soon as my eating habits once again grew erratic.

Anxiety Disorders

Everyone feels periods of anxiety and nervousness, but those people with anxiety disorders suffer from exaggerated worry and tension that is out of proportion with any real threat or problem. Symptoms can be both physical and emotional. Two anxiety disorders that typically predate and accompany anorexia nervosa and/or bulimia nervosa are social phobia (excessive self-consciousness and nervousness in public and/or in social situations) and obsessive-compulsive disorder (OCD; having an obsession about a certain idea and/or feeling compelled by an urgent need to engage in certain behaviors or rituals). Other anxiety disorders that may coexist with eating disorders are generalized anxiety disorder (GAD; excessive worries about everyday events that don't necessarily warrant that much concern) and post-traumatic stress disorder (PTSD; vivid flashbacks and fears about a traumatic event that occurred in the past).

My OCD was diagnosed around the same time as my eating disorder, though I was suffering from the OCD long before the eating disorder. I took great pains to hide my irrational fears and bizarre compulsions from family and friends. Unluckily for me, I was successful. One of my former therapists says that there was a good chance my eating disorder could have been averted with proper diagnosis and early treatment of the OCD. Due to the very ritualistic nature of my eating disorder (constant calorie counting of *everything* that passed my lips, rigid rules about what to eat and drink, obsessive weighing rituals, and so on), both my current treatment team and I believe that my experiences with anorexia and bulimia are almost certainly an extension of my OCD.

... there was a good chance my eating disorder could have been averted with proper diagnosis and early treatment of the OCD.

Now that I am on the proper medications, have received appropriate behavioral therapies for the bipolar depression and OCD, and am eating much better, I feel completely different, and am much better equipped to remain in recovery from my eating disorder.

Substance Use Disorders

The misuse of substances like alcohol and drugs is seen in increased numbers in individuals with eating disorders, especially those with bulimia nervosa and with the binge/purge subtype of anorexia nervosa. In both anorexia and bulimia, the substance abuse tends to begin after the onset of the eating disorder, and can include the use of alcohol, marijuana, and cocaine.

Diagnostic Migration

Another factor that can complicate the diagnosis and treatment of an eating disorder is something clinicians call "diagnostic migration," which is the shift of an individual's illness across diagnostic categories from one eating disorder or subtype to another. Some people's diagnoses may migrate from bulimia nervosa to anorexia nervosa, but the most frequent change is from the restricting subtype of anorexia nervosa to the binge/purge subtype or to bulimia nervosa. In one study, reported in 2002, more than 50% of people with the restricting subtype of anorexia nervosa, both adolescents and adults, developed bulimic symptoms. Currently, scientists remain unsure what factors lead to the development of bulimic symptoms in persons with the restricting subtype of anorexia nervosa, or what the timeline of this development is.

I began to develop symptoms of bulimia as I was attempting to recover from anorexia. Part of what led to the binge eating was the long, extreme time of food deprivation, as well as medications that I needed for other conditions, like depression and bipolar disorder, which rapidly increased my appetite. The medications also caused nausea, leading me to begin vomiting from physiological reasons. However, I began to force myself to vomit even after the nausea passed, out of fear of weight gain. This started a vicious cycle that ended up in almost daily binge eating and purging.

So, What Next?

If you are anything like me, you will have read through these pages and thought, "Yeah, and . . . ?" The information you've just read is important, but the crucial issue is how it applies to you. If you think you may be experiencing the effects of an eating disorder, my advice is this: Go to a doctor and get it checked out. The worst that can happen is that you find out nothing is wrong. (By the way, if you're not honest about *all* of your symptoms, an all-clear from your physician doesn't mean a whole lot. Been there, done that.) Knowing exactly what *is* wrong can help you determine how best to begin recovery.

An eating disorder may tell you many false and unkind things: that you're not sick enough to get help, that you don't deserve help, that you can fix it yourself, that everyone will think you're a freak if you reveal your behaviors—maybe even that you don't have a problem at all.

An eating disorder may tell you many false and unkind things . . .

What is hard to comprehend about eating disorders, especially for sufferers, is that problems can arise very quickly, and the disorder can suck you in even faster. I fell from virtually normal into severe restricting and overexercise in a matter of *weeks*. Getting treatment for an eating disorder as early as possible is the best way to ensure that you will get better faster and stay healthy for good. One of my biggest regrets is that I didn't do anything about my problem when it first surfaced, and instead deliberately ignored the concerns of friends and family.

Chapter Four

After the Diagnosis: Getting the Right Treatment for You

S o someone has told you that you have an eating disorder. That person may be a parent or a friend. Maybe it's an internist, pediatrician, therapist, or dietician. Maybe it's another caring person in your life. Maybe you didn't need anyone to tell you, but know already that something is very wrong.

My parents were telling me for months that I wasn't eating right and that I was getting increasingly obstinate and thin. Regardless of who expressed concerns about my eating habits and weight, I supplied plenty of ammunition to the contrary. Even when I began to realize that my eating and exercise habits weren't supporting the life I wanted to lead, I still believed I was in full control of what I was doing. My eating disorder told me I wasn't thin enough to have anorexia. Ed said that if there was anyone in the world who was thinner than I, I couldn't be anorexic. My periods hadn't stopped. I binged and purged occasionally, but not enough to meet the criteria for bulimia. Even when I was desperately ill and in the emergency room for the third time in

> *My eating disorder told me I wasn't thin enough to have anorexia.*

a week, I still didn't believe I had an eating disorder. I grew huffy and pissy every time my parents brought up the subject of food and eating. There was *nothing* wrong with me. What were they talking about? Didn't they trust me? It's obvious now that they had good reason to be concerned, and my eating disorder had good reason to be defensive.

Only now am I beginning to accept that I have a life-threatening illness.

That is what eating disorders are, after all: deadly serious psychiatric illnesses. They are not just a cry for attention. They are not a phase, and you will not just grow out of it. You are never too old or too young to develop an eating disorder. You didn't think your way into it, and you can't think your way out of it. You have to start eating properly to maintain a healthy weight, and stop binge eating and purging behaviors. This is the only way I know of to recover—but you will need a lot of help from others along the way.

Seeking Help

Deciding to seek help for an eating disorder can be extremely difficult and even distressing. It was hard for me to comprehend in my malnourished state that something was wrong. I also had intense fears of people seeing me as less than perfect. My greatest fear was that any sort of treatment would make me gain ridiculous amounts of weight, which was the most horrific, frightening thing I could possibly imagine. I would have to give up my eating and exercise rituals, which were the only way I knew how to ratchet down the intolerable anxiety that ruled my life. It wasn't that I didn't *want* to seek help; I very much did. I was simply too frightened of the consequences of eating to face a plate of food.

A brief caveat before I discuss professional treatment: Not all health professionals are created equal. Some doctors have essentially no expertise in eating disorders and wouldn't recognize one if it hit them in the face with a brick. When you talk to your doctor about your concerns, subtlety isn't the way to go. I have outright told some physicians that I had anorexia, and they still said that I was full of crap. (Although, having been starving myself and purging, I can assure you that was not the case.) I used the brick-in-the-face method at an urgent care clinic, meeting all the criteria for anorexia nervosa, and was told I only had a thyroid problem and that, at age 20, I was too old to have an eating disorder. If you think that you have an eating disorder but your doctor won't listen to you, find one who will. The best bet is to find a general practitioner (such as a pediatrician or internist) or, even better, an eating disorder specialist. Hospitals and college health centers can often give you good names and assist you on your search, even if you're not officially a patient or student there.

> If you think that you have an eating disorder but your doctor won't listen to you, find one who will.

Once you find a qualified physician, he or she will examine you to make sure there are no overwhelming medical issues that need to be addressed before you start treatment. Most commonly, your doctor will ask you about your current eating behaviors, check your weight, blood pressure, and pulse, perform an electrocardiogram (EKG) to check for cardiac abnormalities, and do blood tests to make sure you have proper levels of electrolytes, blood sugar, disease-fighting white blood cells, and iron. This can typically be done during one visit, with a follow-up to discuss the results.

When I was first diagnosed, I saw my doctor once a week for a weigh-in and a check of my vital signs. My doctor also helped me understand the many medical complications caused by my eating disorder, such as dehydration, low pulse and blood pressure, and the growth of lanugo all over my body. She explained that many of the psychological problems I was having, such as depression and anxiety, would lessen once I began to eat properly. I still see my internist regularly now that I am in recovery; she continues to monitor my weight, blood pressure, and pulse.

Since my eating disorder had lasted for many years, I developed chronic medical issues that require specialist care. Your primary care doctor is a good person to ask for referrals to the other specialists you may need to see. In addition, there are a number of professional psychiatric or psychological organizations and mental health associations that can offer assistance and referrals for mental health providers in your area (for a list of some of these groups and their contact information, see the Resources section of this book). You or your parents should also contact your insurance carrier for a referral; this will most likely ensure that your treatment will be at least partially covered under your insurance policy.

Goals of Treatment

While the goals of complete recovery include both physical and mental healing, often priorities need to be made as to what areas to tackle first. Several important goals to achieve, in order of decreasing urgency, include:

1. Correct potentially life-threatening health complications (such as heart irregularities, low blood pressure, and dehydration)

2. Minimize risks of self-harm, such as suicidal behavior
3. Restore weight to normal
4. Develop normal eating behavior and eliminate binge eating and purging
5. Address psychological and psychosocial issues (such as low self-esteem, body image distortion, and problems in interpersonal relationships)
6. Maintain long-term recovery

Starting Treatment

Once you get a comprehensive evaluation from your physician to assess your physical and mental well being, you will move on to more specific forms of therapy. Indeed, after you've gotten the diagnosis, the best way to combat your eating disorder is to fight it on multiple fronts. You may, for example, start on an outpatient basis by seeing a psychotherapist or a psychiatrist and perhaps a dietician, as well as your physician for medical monitoring.

You will see your treatment team quite often as you begin to recover from your eating disorder. Depending on your needs, you may see your therapist and dietician as much as two or three times a week. As you become more solid in recovery, you can step down to once a week or twice monthly appointments. For most of my time in recovery, I saw my therapist and dietician once a week, and increased the frequency when I struggled.

As well, friends and family should be involved in your efforts to recover. Often, your family will be your first line of defense against your eating disorder. In other cases, it may be that your friends will be involved as much, or even more than, your family. For me, the assistance of my parents was crucial to recovery. When I wasn't living at home, I sometimes had

Your Treatment Team, Communication, and You

Once you have assembled a team of professionals to help you fight your eating disorder, they can best be utilized if they communicate with one another regularly. I have found this to be crucial, because if everyone is not on the same page, the conflicting messages can be confusing and damaging. In order to make this communication possible, you will be asked to sign a release form to allow all of your care providers to talk freely.

"virtual dinners" with my mom, where we would both eat and chat on the phone at the same time, which helped me commit to eating and maintaining a focus on nourishing my body. I could call my mom at any hour of the day and receive consistent, loving support. My friends also helped keep me centered by responding to my e-mails and taking me out for coffee when I became too obsessed with food and weight. Whatever the circumstances, it is important to understand that an eating dis-

... it is important to understand that an eating disorder cannot be conquered by you alone.

order cannot be conquered by you alone. I've never met a person who successfully recovered without some sort of outside help, whether professional or not.

But sometimes that outside help may not be totally effective for you as an outpatient, and you may need a more aggressive treatment plan through, say, an inpatient program or a residential treatment facility that can better stabilize you medically and psychiatrically. I will discuss these settings a bit later in the chapter, but first let's take a close look at a few of the treatment providers you might encounter in any setting, and what they can do for you.

Close-up on the Treatment Team:
Who They Are and What They Can Do for You

The Dietician

In books about eating disorders, the words "dietician" and "nutritionist" tend to be used interchangeably. While there are many similarities, there are significant differences between the two labels. Anyone can call him or herself a "nutritionist"; there are no laws governing the usage of this title. However, one must complete an internship and pass a comprehensive exam administered by the American Dietetic Association in order to call oneself a "registered dietician." I would advise caution in seeing a nutritionist who is not a registered dietician (RD), because there is otherwise no way to ensure that he or she has received the proper training to be advising you on nutrition.

When I first began treatment for anorexia, I thought the entire purpose of a dietician was to make me fat. She was The Enemy, to be fought with every resource my eating disorder and I could muster.

I was rather mistaken about this.

My dietician has been a key player on my road to recovery. She helped me better understand and conquer my food rituals and anxieties so that I could begin to adequately nourish my body. She never judged me for slipping up, or when I confessed behaviors I found shameful and embarrassing. Together, we developed a food plan that both worked for me and would restore me to a healthy weight. Her goals were *never* to "fatten me up," as much as my eating disorder tried to convince me of this. We worked together so that I would achieve optimum health. Food is now one of the medicines I take on a daily basis to keep myself in recovery from my eating disorder. I continue to see my dietician regularly to help me fine-tune my eating habits depending on my current living and working situations.

I found it helpful to keep my parents updated on my current meal plan so that they could hold me accountable, especially when I was living at home. As I moved out and began living on my own, they naturally became less involved, but the line of communication between my parents and my dietician remained open. How an individual's parents will be involved with this nutrition therapy will vary from person to person and from dietician to dietician. At times, your parents may be advised to oversee all of your food choices in order to help you battle your eating disorder.

While it is sometimes difficult to obtain insurance coverage for seeing a dietician, a written prescription from your primary care physician might sway your insurance company to cover these services. Some insurance companies do cover visits to a dietician, as long as you see one they've pre-approved, so check your insurer's Web site. Many dieticians offer sliding scales, based on your family's ability to pay, if no insurance coverage is available. Even occasional sessions with a dietician can be very helpful in aiding your recovery.

The Psychotherapist

I have seen several different psychotherapists over the years, each of whom has helped me through my different stages of recovery. While a therapist who specializes in eating disorders is best, one who is knowledgeable of the area and has a philosophy you can work with is also a good bet.

There are several kinds of mental health professionals who practice psychotherapy (also known as talk therapy). A psychiatrist is a medical doctor who specializes in the diagnosis and treatment of mental illnesses and emotional problems. Psychiatrists can prescribe medications as well as provide psychotherapy, and will have an M.D. after their name. A clinical psychologist also specializes in mental illness, and has a doctorate (Ph.D. or Psy.D.), typically in psychology, but usually cannot prescribe drugs. A social worker (usually an M.S.W. or LIC.S.W.) has obtained a master's degree, typically takes a broad approach to counseling about issues at home, and even at school, and does not prescribe drugs. Which type of psychotherapist you see will depend on a number of factors, including the availability of practitioners in your area, your particular experiences with your illness, your insurance coverage, and more. Oftentimes people with eating disorders and other illnesses will see a psychiatrist to monitor any medication they are taking (more on this later) as well as a psychotherapist for psychotherapy.

Sometimes, your ability to see a therapist you like and work well with may be limited by insurance coverage, both of the specific therapist and by the number of visits allowed per year by insurance plans. While this is very difficult and frustrating, there are ways around the problem. Many therapists work on a sliding scale, which means that their fee is based on your ability to pay. As well, if your therapist has you on a solid path to recovery, it may be worth the cost to you and your family to continue with that therapist even without insurance coverage. Lastly, your therapist may be able to advocate for you with the insurance company to help extend your coverage.

In general, psychotherapy for your eating disorder can help you learn the skills and gain the knowledge that you will need in order to recover. It can help you to understand the origins of your eating disorder, identify and change self-defeating ways of thinking, improve interpersonal relationships, learn how to respond to difficult situations without lapsing into disordered eating, and rebuild your life as you move into recovery. It's a pretty large task for anyone, and so there are a variety of therapies that are used to treat an eating disorder. I have used bits and pieces of each of the therapies described below, and, while all of them have helped me, some have been more effective for me than others. The important thing is to find an approach that works best for *you*. There is no right or wrong answer.

The important thing is to find an approach that works best for you. There is no right or wrong answer.

Because of this, there are very few studies that can effectively "prove" which treatments work best, especially in adolescents and young people. There are some ongoing studies that are trying to gather concrete evidence as to which approach is the most effective, but at the moment, many of the recommendations are based on a limited amount of research and the advice

---

Good Questions to Ask Your Therapist:

- What is your general approach to treatment? What will be the process of therapy as time goes on?
- Do you accept my family's insurance plan?
- How often do I need to make appointments with you?
- What are your policies on contacting you after-hours?
- How will you involve my family in my recovery?
- What information will you keep confidential, and what will you share with my parents?
- What will you do should I become medically unstable?
- How will you work with any other members of my treatment team?
- What are your views on the use of psychiatric medications?

There are no right or wrong answers to these questions. Sometimes, the best therapist is one with whom you feel the most comfortable and can be totally honest about all of your thoughts and behaviors. Talk to your therapist and your parents to make a decision with which everyone is satisfied.

(Some information courtesy National Eating Disorders Association)

of specialists. However, if a somewhat "unconventional" approach seems to work for you, then go with it. You can always change your mind later and find another way that will help you along this section of your road to recovery.

INDIVIDUAL PSYCHOTHERAPY

Individual psychotherapy is a private, one-on-one treatment that occurs between a trained psychotherapist and a patient, usually once or twice a week. You will likely continue school with minimal or no interruptions, though after-school activities may need adjustment. There are several different kinds of individual psychotherapy, which I'll discuss below.

When I was first advised to see a therapist for depression and OCD in college, I had nightmares of couches and some bearded German doctor in spectacles peering at me and asking me about my mother. Thankfully, it was nothing like that. Mostly, I have sat in a chair. I have had therapy in an office and in a house. None of my therapists have had beards—though that was likely because they were all women.

I first thought it ludicrous, that an hour in a therapist's office could cure me of my eating disorder. I was right—it didn't. And it's very unlikely that just one hour a week will cure you, either. In order to recover, I found I had to take therapy *out of the office*. I had to *live* what I was learning. When my therapist told me to be gentle with myself, nodding in agreement wasn't enough. I had to actually start treating myself with respect and kindness.

In order to recover, I found I had to take therapy out of the office. I had to live what I was learning.

Therapy can be difficult and grueling, and sometimes the mental distress can get worse before it gets better. The eating disorder does not like to be challenged, nor does it like its secrets revealed. However, a therapist can be crucial in providing support to both stop the symptoms of your eating disorder and to help work through any harmful thinking patterns.

There are numerous psychological approaches that a therapist may work from, though the majority of therapists combine several different approaches, which are discussed below.

Psychodynamically Oriented, Supportive Psychotherapy

Although there are no data available on success rates, this type of individual therapy is the approach most commonly employed in the treatment of any type of psychological problem, including an eating disorder. This approach is traditionally associated with the ideas of Sigmund Freud, but it has branched out to include many different methods. The common thread is a focus on a person's inner psychological experience and the belief that unresolved issues from childhood are fueling the current problems. The therapy focuses on resolving these conflicts to allow a person to function more effectively.

What makes this form of therapy especially useful for someone with an eating disorder is that it creates a safe space in which he or she can freely share feelings without worrying about who might approve or disapprove of what is being said. Throughout my entire life, I would remain silent and keep all of my distressing feelings to myself for fear of saying the wrong thing or admitting that I wasn't as perfect as everyone thought I was. As I came to trust my therapist with facts or feelings I found shameful, and have her invite me back to her office the next week despite my fears of rejection, I realized that she was not going to judge me. "Pain," says my therapist, "is what brings people closer together." To be sure, it took quite some time for me to warm up to my therapist, let alone begin to trust her.

I didn't even initially like her, only to find after several appointments that we made a good team at fighting the eating disorder.

Of course, talking to a stranger about very personal information freely and immediately is nearly impossible, regardless of the letters that may appear after their name. It may take several sessions to begin to open up to your therapist. My eating disorder very loudly told me to lie about what I was eating and how I was feeling. My head felt like it was going to explode because all of the infighting that developed as my wise mind began to duel with my eating disorder. I found that getting angry at my therapist was a good sign that she had found an area on which I needed to work. My first therapist told me that she knew she had hit pay dirt when I began to scream at her for being a blabbering idiot. My eating disorder didn't want me working on this problem because it meant I would divest him of power. I usually came back the next week and sheepishly apologized. She recognized that my eating disorder was yelling at her, not me.

My eating disorder didn't want me working on this problem because it meant I would divest him of power.

Therapy was also a good place for me to learn how to express myself without resorting to eating disordered behaviors. I found that not eating was a profound way for me to express myself and my feelings without having to use my voice. It removed any shame I felt about being inadequate and burdening other people with my problems. "Carrie! Use your words!" my former therapist used to urge me. I still struggle with this, but knowing that I will sit in an office for an hour with someone who doesn't judge me gives me the opportunity to speak my mind. Even discussing your fears about expressing yourself can help you better understand the origins of this problem and work through it.

I spent years discussing my history and issues I thought contributed to my eating disorder, yet only minimal progress was made toward decreasing my eating disorder symptoms. I could understand why I might have fallen victim to an eating disorder, but I didn't know what to do about it when in the midst of a particularly brutal struggle. In fact, the more I have learned how to respond to my eating disorder, the more I understand that there is no clear reason *why* I developed anorexia and bulimia. And that I *can* recover without answering that question.

As I got stronger in my recovery, I developed terrible, haunting fears that the second I was not starving, binge eating, or purging, my treatment team would drop me. So I greatly resisted giving up my eating disordered behaviors because they were the only way I knew how to communicate that my life wasn't okay, that *I* wasn't okay. What therapy taught me was how to use my voice to communicate my needs. I began to understand that the only way people would know I was struggling was to actively tell them.

Interpersonal Psychotherapy

Interpersonal psychotherapy, abbreviated as IPT, is similar to psychodynamic therapy, but differs in several important aspects. IPT is a short-term therapy that runs from 12 to 16 sessions, and was developed as a treatment for depression among adults, focusing on improving social functioning. The therapist is quite active in helping you identify problem areas, such as "role transitions," and uses several specific techniques, such as role playing, to help you develop new methods of dealing with your interpersonal relationships.

Initially developed and tested in adults with very positive results, IPT has been adapted for use in adolescents, focusing on areas important to young people, such as separation from parents, sexual relationships, and peer pressures. These are areas in which people with eating disorders frequently struggle. IPT is also effective in treating the depression that frequently accompanies an eating disorder.

Cognitive-Behavioral Therapy

Cognitive-behavioral therapy (CBT) was originally developed for adults with depression in the 1960s and is based on the theory that persistent but unhealthy thinking patterns are key contributors to emotional disturbances. There is evidence that supports the effectiveness of CBT for treating depression and anxiety disorders, and beginning in the 1970s it was tailored specifically for the treatment of eating disorders.

As the name implies, CBT focuses on "cognition" (one's views and perceptions of oneself) and "behavior" (one's reactions to those perceptions), with the aim of correcting those ingrained patterns of cognition and behavior that may be contributing to one's illness. The cognitive part of CBT helps you identify unrealistic thoughts and/or habitually pessimistic attitudes and then reframe them in more realistic or optimistic terms. The behavioral part of CBT helps you to change the way you react to the world around you by developing better coping strategies for dealing with your interpersonal relationships and your illness.

The primary importance of CBT in treating an eating disorder lies in its exploration of your idealized body weight and shape and of your behavioral responses to that idealization. My dietician utilized this approach in her work with me, and had me record the thoughts that preceded my eating disorder behaviors and then form a more realistic view of the situation. As well, when I entered a starving–binge eating–purging cycle, she helped me understand that the binge eating was triggered by the restricting, and the best way to stop a binge was to stop the restricting. Then, if a binge did occur, I learned that although purging momentarily relieved the shame and anxiety I felt about binge eating, it created more shame in the long run. I also learned how to change my views on a proper body size and shape for myself, in order to alter my behaviors that chased those thoughts.

CBT also involves "homework," such as keeping a food and feelings log, eating previously "forbidden" foods, and developing skills for coping with high-risk situations that might lead to food restriction, binge eating, and/or purging. These skills are also used to help prevent a relapse at the conclusion of treatment.

Dialectical-Behavioral Therapy

Dialectical-behavioral therapy (DBT) was developed in the early 1990s as a treatment for borderline personality disorder, a mental illness characterized by severe instability of moods, interpersonal relationships, self-image, and behavior. DBT consists of four different modules: mindfulness, interpersonal effectiveness, distress tolerance, and emotion regulation. Many times, DBT is used as both individual therapy and as group therapy (I'll discuss group therapy in more detail later in this chapter). The four modules are taught in a weekly two-hour group therapy session, and the skills are practiced at a weekly individual therapy session. DBT typically lasts for approximately one year, during which the skills are taught and practiced.

DBT is similar to cognitive-behavioral therapy in that thoughts and actions are separated. The difference between the two therapies is that CBT encourages you to change thoughts before you change your behaviors; DBT works the exact opposite way. I have participated in DBT group therapy while in residential treatment, and the therapist's favorite saying was

"Feelings chase behaviors." When I had fears of wearing a bathing suit in public, I didn't try to talk myself into believing that everyone wasn't thinking I was fat. Instead, I started wearing a bathing suit for short time periods in order to expe-

... the therapist's favorite saying was "Feelings chase behaviors."

rience the fact that I wouldn't die and other people wouldn't flee from the sight of me in spandex. Unless I had experienced wearing a bathing suit, I would have never stopped being afraid of it.

So You Want to See a Different Therapist...

As I began recovery after discharge from inpatient treatment, I found a therapist who was very strict about helping me get back to and maintain a healthy weight. However, we spent so much time talking about my past that I never quite learned how to tackle my current issues. It helped to learn my triggers and the problems that had contributed to the development of my eating disorder, but I needed to start learning solutions. After butting heads a few too many times, I decided to start seeing a different therapist. My old therapist gave me referrals to other eating disorder specialists in the area, and I began the interview process. The new therapist was more behaviorally based and helped me to identify my very self-defeating ways of thinking and ways to keep me on track in recovery. All of the different therapists I have seen over the years have played an influential role on helping me to recovery.

If you have been working with a therapist for a while, even if you feel a good connection with him or her, and haven't made any noticeable progress toward decreasing your eating disorder behaviors, it might be time to look into other therapists. A good therapist will be able to determine whether he or she thinks that the two of you will make a good team, and also when it might be time to move on.

It is possible that you and your therapist simply don't have the same ideas about your therapy, or that your personalities don't mesh quite right. Whatever the reason, if you decide that you'd like to work with a new therapist, don't be shy in considering this option. Just be sure to ask yourself whether it's the therapist you don't like—or the therapy itself.

FAMILY THERAPY

In addition to individual psychotherapy, other approaches have been used in the treatment of eating disorders. One such approach is family therapy, which recent research has shown can be effective in helping to treat anorexia nervosa, and possibly also bulimia nervosa. Even if you are in individual treatment, your psychotherapist might recommend that your family be involved in some of your therapy sessions, because it can be extremely useful in helping your parents to understand your eating disorder and the difficulties that you are going through, as well as to learn how to support you in your recovery. Siblings can benefit from participation in family therapy, as they are affected by the eating disorder too, and may be confused and worried about you. The overall goals of treatment in family therapy include identifying harmful patterns that may contribute to or arise from the eating disorder, opening lines of communication, teaching coping skills, strengthening family bonds, reducing conflict, and increasing empathy among family members.

Even when I wasn't living at home, I participated in family therapy because it was still of immense value in helping my parents and me communicate better about all of our needs. Living at home during a brief period after I developed my eating disorder, both my family and I found working with a family therapist to be infinitely helpful in managing the stress of living with an eating disordered person.

The Maudsley Method

Named for the hospital in London where it was developed, this form of family therapy focuses less on the psychological roots of disordered eating and more on addressing actual eating problems and behavior. The participation of the family is vital to the Maudsley method because parents will initially be responsible for ensuring that you eat properly and reach a healthier weight. Food and its role in the family dynamic are examined in therapy, as are the effects the eating disorder has on everyone. Each member of the family cooperates to support you in reaching a goal weight set by the doctor. Once your weight is restored, treatment begins to focus more on family and individual concerns, and the therapist will provide problem-solving skills to help prevent the recurrence of the eating disorder.

The Maudsley method was developed to treat anorexia nervosa, but experts are now beginning to apply it to bulimia nervosa as well. As you can probably imagine, this particular type of family therapy isn't for everyone—you may not be living at home, or you may have reason to believe that your family should not take such an active role in your recovery. But the method has been successful for many families, so it's worth knowing it's an option.

GROUP THERAPY

In group therapy, a mental health care professional facilitates a dialogue among people trying to recover from similar diseases. For those suffering from eating disorders, a group discussion might focus on body image issues, the importance of food, social problems, family conflicts, and so on. Group therapy sessions usually take place in intensive treatment programs (which are discussed at length later in this chapter).

The Psychiatrist

In addition to psychotherapeutic approaches to combating your eating disorder, you may also be prescribed psychotropic medication by a psychiatrist. As previously mentioned, psychiatrists are medical doctors (M.D.s) who specialize in treating mental illness. Not only might they provide psychotherapy, but they are also licensed to prescribe and monitor medications for mood disorders, anxiety disorders, and other mental conditions.

PSYCHIATRIC MEDICATIONS

The psychiatric medications most frequently prescribed to help treat eating disorders are antidepressants, although the only antidepressant officially approved by the Food and Drug Administration (FDA) to treat an eating disorder is fluoxetine (Prozac)—for bulimia nervosa. Fluoxetine is a member of a class of drugs known as selective serotonin reuptake inhibitors (SSRIs) including sertraline (Zoloft), citalopram (Celexa), and several others. Only fluoxetine has been extensively studied in the treatment of eating disorders—hence, its FDA approval. Physicians sometimes decide to recommend other antidepressants because of small differences between fluoxetine and the other SSRIs, and this is entirely in accordance with FDA regulations.

Surprisingly, while antidepressants have been demonstrated convincingly to be effective in the treatment of bulimia nervosa, neither fluoxetine nor other antidepressants appear to be especially helpful for anorexia nervosa, either when patients are underweight or immediately after they regain weight and are attempting to stay well. Researchers believe that the malnutrition inherent in anorexia in particular may interfere with the therapeutic action of antidepressants.

Some ongoing research suggests that another group of medications known as the *atypical antipsychotics* might be helpful in treating anorexia. These drugs are usually prescribed for people suffering from schizophrenia or bipolar disorder, but one in particular, olanzapine (Zyprexa), has shown promise in some studies of providing benefit for children, adolescents, and adults with anorexia nervosa. Psychiatric medications may cause unwanted side effects or allergic reactions, so it is important to talk to your doctor about these, and you should be closely monitored by your doctor whenever you start a new drug.

It's important to note that most medications your psychiatrist might recommend have not been proven to be effective in children and adolescents. This doesn't mean that they won't work—just that not enough research has been done yet to show for sure that they *will*. Some of the biological factors inherent in children and adolescents, such as still-developing brains and shifting hormone levels, may impact the effectiveness of psychiatric medications. Also, you should keep close tabs on any and all symptoms that you experience while taking a new medication. Particularly when your body is weakened by an eating disorder, the introduction of drugs to your system can have unexpected consequences—for instance, cardiac abnormalities often associated with anorexia could make the use of certain antidepressants more risky.

... you should keep close tabs on any and all symptoms that you experience while taking a new medication.

Of course, many young people are able to successfully recover from their eating disorder without the use of psychiatric medications, but if your treatment team recommends that you try taking one, you may find that it provides the extra boost you need to stay in recovery. Discuss the pros and cons of taking medication with your doctor and with your family. Carefully monitor your health while on these medications and be sure to tell someone immediately if you start to experience new symptoms.

Starting an antidepressant or other psychiatric medication can be scary, but I found my body needed certain medications

FDA "Black Box" Label Warning on Antidepressant Drugs

In October 2004, the U.S. Food and Drug Administration (FDA) issued a Public Health Advisory about the increased risk of suicidal thoughts and behavior ("suicidality") in children and adolescents being treated with selective serotonin reuptake inhibitors (SSRIs). As part of its report, the agency directed the manufacturers not only of SSRIs but of *all* antidepressant medications to add a "black box" label warning health professionals about the increased risk of suicidality in children and adolescents who are prescribed these medications. This revised labeling is based on studies of five SSRIs—including citalopram (Celexa), fluoxetine (Prozac), fluvoxamine (Luvox), paroxetine (Paxil), and sertraline (Zoloft)—as well as four "atypical" antidepressants: bupropion (Wellbutrin), mirtazapine (Remeron), nefazodone (Serzone), and venlafaxine (Effexor XR).

What this all means is that the use of some psychiatric medications by some children and adolescents may possibly increase their thoughts about suicide. If you are prescribed *any* medication it is extremely important that you be open and honest with your doctor about new symptoms. If you begin to experience suicidal thoughts, or become more depressed, tell your therapist or psychiatrist right away. If you can't get in touch with them immediately, tell a parent or trusted friend what you are experiencing.

The American Academy of Child and Adolescent Psychiatry has provided a useful and detailed review of these issues, which can be found on its Web site, www.aacap.org. Information from the FDA can be seen at www.fda.gov.

---

in order to function. If my anxiety and bipolar disorder are not properly managed, I find it almost impossible to remain in recovery. I also try to be diligent about taking my medication consistently, and on time—and you should too. Remember that a medication is only effective if it is taken properly.

Remember that a medication is only effective if it is taken properly.

Intensive Treatment Options

The therapeutic approaches I've been discussing—psychotherapy and medication—are often successful in reversing eating disorder syndromes, and many people are able to recover on an outpatient basis after having committed to psychotherapy alone. However, sometimes a higher level of structure and support is needed to help a person begin to recover. In those cases, inpatient, residential, and day treatment programs can be utilized.

Intensive Outpatient Program (IOP)

An IOP requires patients to come to an outpatient clinic for several hours on several days per week, typically in the evenings. While at the clinic, the patient will attend therapy sessions (usually group therapy) and, in many cases, have supervised meals.

Partial Hospitalization Program (PHP) or Day Hospital Care

A partial hospital program is often recommended for people making a transition back home from an inpatient or residential facility. Lasting from four to eight hours per day (usually Monday through Friday), a PHP provides structured eating situations and active treatment interventions while allowing you to live at home and participate in certain school activities. A PHP may also be recommended as a first intervention if you need close supervision but not the 24-hour care provided in hospital and residential settings.

After a two-week inpatient psychiatric hospital stay, I participated in a partial hospital program for a month, which helped me maintain a healthier weight and learn how to deal with life in more manageable chunks than if I had left the hospital and tried to tackle everything all at once. The dependable structure of being in the clinic for six hours a day also provided me with the psychological support I needed at the time.

Inpatient Psychiatric Hospitalization

Before I was hospitalized on a psych floor for my eating disorder, my images of these places were very much reminiscent of the movie *One Flew Over the Cuckoo's Nest*. This wasn't quite true—although I did meet one nurse who was hauntingly similar to the evil Nurse Ratched. I thought that no one else there would understand an eating disorder. I didn't even think that a person with an eating disorder belonged in a psych ward. However, talking to other patients about their psychological struggles helped me remember that eating disorders are also psychiatric illnesses that need treatment. No one there, including me, *asked* for this illness, but we all needed intense help in overcoming it.

No one there, including me, asked for this illness, but we all needed intense help in overcoming it.

Inpatient psychiatric hospitalization can both stabilize a person medically and begin to help him or her to focus more intensively on behavioral and psychological issues. Most inpatient psychiatric units are located in a general hospital and often provide care to young people with all types of psychiatric problems. Meals are closely supervised, and you may be given intensive individual and/or group therapy. Bathrooms are also usually monitored, meaning someone will watch you while you are in the bathroom and/or shower, and check the toilet when you are finished. This has been the case during most of my times in inpatient treatment, and although embarrassing, it helped me to remember that the staff members who monitored me did this every day. One of the nurse's assistants that worked with me in the hospital reassured me that "It's not like I look in the bowl and think 'Huh. Looks like ya'll had some corn for dinner yesterday.'"

Conditions that may coexist with the eating disorder (such as depression, anxiety disorders, and obsessive-compulsive disorder—see Chapter 3) are carefully assessed, and appropriate treatment initiated. Virtually all inpatient psychiatric units have 24-hour support available from physicians, psychiatrists, psychologists, nurses, and dieticians. Most people stay in an inpatient unit for one to four weeks, although it can be longer or shorter based on your individual needs, as well as your insurance and financial supports.

One common misconception among people with eating disorders, which I've been guilty of as well, is that all people in an inpatient unit for eating disorders are skin and bones. This was not the case, in either of my two inpatient hospitalizations. While some of the people were underweight, many more

---

Hospitalization Without Consent: What Are Your Rights?

If you are under 18, then your parents can sign you into treatment without your consent, and will be required to sign you out of treatment as well. Even after you turn 18, you can still be hospitalized without your consent if your parents or treatment team determine that you are incapable of making your own medical decisions. This is typically done by court order, and can consist of medical guardianship or court-ordered treatment. I have been threatened with this twice during the course of my eating disorder (only one of those times was when I was severely underweight), and the fear of being forced to undergo treatments without my consent was enough to convince me to enter treatment voluntarily.

were of fairly normal weight. Other psychiatric considerations influence the need for hospitalization, such as your ability to combat your eating disorder on an outpatient basis, suicidal thoughts, and other coexisting psychological disorders. Weight is not the only indicator of the seriousness of an eating disorder—you can die from an eating disorder at any weight. People with eating disorders come in all different shapes and sizes, even in an inpatient unit.

Residential Treatment

Residential treatment for an eating disorder is very similar to inpatient psychiatric treatment, except on a smaller scale, and in a more "home-like" environment. Most residential treatment centers do not handle people who are medically unstable, and it is not uncommon to transfer to residential treatment after an inpatient stay. Treatment for adolescents typically includes individual and group therapy, creative therapy (such as art, music, and writing), academic services, nutrition classes, and recreational activities. Most people stay in a residential program for several months, which I have found to be necessary to break the cycle of the eating disorder.

My last treatment experience was at a residential facility, where I lived in a normal home with five other women with eating disorders. I got out in the community frequently enough that I was able to process "real-life" experiences while still in intensive treatment. I ate regular food at regular intervals, and re-learned how much food was really required in order to gain weight. Because I didn't have much of a choice over what I was served and when, I wasn't able to bargain with the eating disorder as to how few calories I could eat. Lastly, the small environment was helpful for me to learn valuable interpersonal and behavioral skills to take with me when I left.

Residential treatment often focuses more on the underlying psychological issues, such as low self-esteem, self-defeating ways of thinking, interpersonal relationship skills, as well as on the stabilization of eating patterns and body weight. While all of this work can be crucial in recovering from an eating disorder, it also means that there has to be quite a bit of self-motivation in order to gain the full benefit of a program. You get out what you put in. Each time I have entered treatment, I have come with more than my fair share of ambivalence. I knew I didn't want my life to be this way; I just wasn't sure I wanted to give up the eating disorder. As I began to eat better and trust my treatment team, I was able to work through much of my ambivalence toward recovery.

As I began to eat better and trust my treatment team, I was able to work through much of my ambivalence toward recovery.

The downside of residential treatment is that it can be quite expensive, and it is not often covered by insurance. As the result of my last seven-month residential stay, both my parents and I have spent a lot of money. The other result is, of course, that I have my life back.

Medical Hospitalization

If your eating disorder has caused severe physical consequences, such as cardiac abnormalities, seizures, or dehydration, short-term hospitalization in a medical unit (even in an intensive care unit) is required to stabilize and then monitor you medically. Vital signs (blood pressure, heart rate, and rhythm) will be watched closely; then the acute physical effects of malnutrition and binge eating and purging will be treated with fluids and medications. If you are underweight or malnourished, you will be re-fed with food, or by intravenous or nasogastric feedings. Hospitalization usually lasts three to ten days, depending on the medical problems and how your body responds to treatment.

Recovery in Any Setting

Recovery from an eating disorder can take a long time, sometimes five or more years. Many times on my road to recovery, I almost threw in the towel because I thought if I hadn't learned the skills right away, then I was destined never to learn them. Apparently, I was just a slow learner. After long-term, intensive treatment, I can function in the world almost like anyone else. I am not yet fully recovered, no, but I am feeling better than I have for years.

Most people I know who have recovered from an eating disorder have done so with outpatient treatment alone, which is often successful in eradicating the eating disorder. However, sometimes people who *do* require inpatient treatment don't get it. For instance, your insurance may not cover the treatment your doctors deem necessary to give you the best shot at recovery. In that case, you may have to evaluate other options, such as the Maudsley method, which is much more economical because it lets you live at home while your parents help normalize your eating habits and re-feed you.

Requiring more intensive therapy, on the other hand, isn't a sign of failure. Many people find they need more than a therapy session or two per week in order to recover. The important thing is not *how* you recover, but instead that you commit to recovery and acknowledge that there will be difficult times ahead. Especially at first, recovery-minded actions

The important thing is not how you recover, but instead that you commit to recovery . . .

will seem foreign and awkward. They require practice and patience. You didn't get sick overnight, and you won't recover overnight. The journey toward recovery—learning new coping skills, and learning how to take care of your body, mind, and spirit—is almost as important as the destination itself.

Chapter Five

The Personal Challenges of Recovery: Practical Tips

R ecovery from an eating disorder can be a long and arduous
process. Many times, I would appear to be thriving on the
outside, yet feel like I was dying on the inside. Or I would have
an upswing, and begin to think that I could conquer my eating
disorder, only to slam back down in a resurgence of symptoms.
Life with an eating disorder *isn't* life. It's about making it
through until tomorrow, when the numbers on the scale will be
down and you will be allowed to eat once more. But then, it's
never enough, and you are right back at square one. I've made
the desperate promises, I've bargained with the eating disorder,
I've sworn I would eat, or that I wouldn't binge and purge, so
many times I have lost count. I have collapsed with exhaustion
for lack of food. I have fallen asleep crying at the side of the
toilet after a night of binge eating and purging. I have come
close to checking out because I couldn't handle my life anymore. It wasn't worth it. But in spite of everything, I have sur-
vived and learned many important lessons along the way.

The focus of this chapter isn't to tell you how to live *with*
an eating disorder. It's to help you make it through the emotional and mental challenges of the recovery process with as little

damage as possible, and to teach you some personal, day-to-day strategies to get and stay healthy. Not every strategy will work for every person, but take what you can use and leave the rest.

Accepting That YOU Have an Eating Disorder

Acceptance of your illness is very important. If you are anything like me, then you might be unsure whether or not you even have an eating disorder. You may not think there is a problem—after all, your weight control strategies could be working. Purging after binge eating might be preventing weight gain. Restricting and over exercising may be causing the weight loss you desire. What on earth could be wrong? I thought these same things many times. Even when my physical condition made it obvious that something was wrong with me, I could not understand the seriousness of the eating disorder. The exhilaration I experienced from weight loss and/or purging, combined with my starving brain, wouldn't allow any sense to get through the concrete wall built by the eating disorder. It took a lot of time and therapy to convince me that I was seriously ill. Since you can't get better until you recognize that you are sick, facing the fact that you may have an eating disorder is a critical first step toward saving your life.

... facing the fact that you may have an eating disorder is a critical first step toward saving your life.

Strategies and Techniques for Maintaining Recovery

The easiest way for me to move through recovery was to break it down into manageable bites—no pun intended. So instead of saying I would eat all of my food for the week, I concentrated on taking one meal at a time. Since I love traveling, I stopped planning trips a year from now and hoping it would carry me through. Instead, I began to read travel books at the library or bookstore, look at trip ideas every week, and subscribe to travel newsletters; I even renewed my passport. I also tried to quit calorie counting "for good," but that never worked. I decided to give myself small rewards for each week I didn't count calories. Immediate rewards work better than long-term payoffs. They can be concrete evidence of the progress you are making. What follows are some other methods I used to get through this difficult process.

Learning to Take Baby Steps

The Great Pyramids in Egypt were not brought down from Mars fully assembled. They had to be shaped, and then dragged into place. Engineering had to be refined to complete these tasks. And man didn't "just" land on the moon. We had to develop the technology, the astronauts had to go through lots of training, engineers had to build the spaceship, get it out on the launch pad, get it into the air, pilots had to make it to the moon and land. Only by completing all of those much smaller steps was the final product possible. The same is true of recovery from an eating disorder.

In the hilariously funny movie *What About Bob?* a psychiatrist writes a book called *Baby Steps* and his obsessive-compulsive patient, played by Bill Murray, takes the concept rather literally. For me, a baby step was buying a scary food at the store, even if I knew I wouldn't be able to eat it right away. Another baby step was doing all of my nighttime cleaning rituals, only in the opposite order in which I usually performed them. I bought half percent milk, then one percent, and finally two percent milk, which is what I drink today. In total, those steps would

have been way too much for me to handle, but each one sepa-
rately was enough of a challenge to push me forward—just not
so much that I would fall over.

Assembling Your Own Personal Cheerleading Squad

The longer I spent with my eating disorder, the more my friends
drifted away. I didn't have the energy or desire to nurture these
relationships; my eating disorder was all that mattered. When I
moved from place to place, I didn't bother to start any new
relationships. Therefore, I found myself with few immediate
friends. Beginning new relationships was really scary for me—
what if people didn't like me? What if they thought I was crazy?
I didn't want to put all of that effort in for no payoff. In my
eyes, relationships should have come with a money-back guarantee. (The problem is that only things like aluminum siding
come with such guarantees.) I realize now that not maintaining friendships was one of the best ways to ensure that my eating disorder remained strong.

I've said it before and I'll say it again: The help of family and
friends is crucial. Friends can help keep you accountable, and
provide a human connection that life with an eating disorder
can often lack. Eventually, you will have to take the steps to recover on your own, but getting that extra boost from someone
or something else is also important. When I got out of treatment,
I planned a short weekend trip with my parents to encourage me
to keep eating. I scheduled regular lunch and dinner dates with
friends who knew about my eating disorder and wouldn't let
me order a garden salad and call it a meal. I kept in close contact
with my therapist and dietician for extra support when I found
myself getting on shaky ground. I know that if my recovery had
been just up to me, I never would have made it.

My psychiatrist tells me that "connection is the cure." Classes through your city or county's continuing education programs can provide an easy way to meet people with similar interests. Joining a club at college is also a great way to meet new people. You can even start a study group or something similar. I have met almost all of my long-term friends this way.

There are some online bulletin boards that can provide virtual support. I only recommend moderated ones that edit out any negative and triggering posts. The best one is through the Something Fishy Web site on Eating Disorders (see Resources). Not only is it moderated, but numbers are not allowed (including weight, BMI, or clothing sizes). It is a great way to feel connected to people struggling with similar issues.

Disclaimer: None of my support people ever obtained a pair of pom-poms or wore a short polyester skirt to help me along my path to recovery. They did not S-P-E-L-L out words of encouragement. They especially did not throw each other up in the air and clap. But even at the moments when they did nothing active, just knowing they were there helped tremendously. Even if none of them had pom-poms.

Urge Surfing

One of my friends aptly named getting through an eating disorder urge as going "urge surfing." Emotions rise in you in waves—building, building, building . . . and then they crash and the waters are still again. Going surfing is scary. When I learned how to bodysurf as a child, I got dunked more than I would end up sliding onto the shore. A noseful of salt water is never fun, but the rewards of coasting into sand are immense. Similarly, riding out scary and painful emotions can be intense, but unless you ride them out and don't bail halfway through, you'll never have the pleasure of moving effortlessly along the water and enjoying the ride, nor the confidence of knowing that you *can* resist harmful urges.

Now where's that cabana boy . . . ?

Exploring New Hobbies

As I began to recover from my eating disorder, I found I had lots of time on my hands that was previously spent obsessing about food, exercising, or binge eating and purging. The loss of what to do sent me fleeing more than once back to the arms of my eating disorder.

What I have found is that expanding your world to include things outside of eating disorder behaviors is crucial. Since I love a good challenge, I began to take up new hobbies as a way to distract myself from the anxiety I felt after eating, as well as to fill the hours that would otherwise have been occupied by the eating disorder. I started with one or two types of crafts, such as crocheting hats and scarves for all my friends (even those who lived in the tropics), and branched out from there. I played endless games of Solitaire on my laptop, and completed books and books of crossword puzzles. Maybe this isn't exactly central to what you might think of as recovery, but it did clear enough of my mind out that I could concentrate on eating and the work I was doing in therapy. Hobbies can help us get through some of the toughest times in life.

. . . expanding your world to include things outside of eating disorder behaviors is crucial.

Not only do new hobbies provide passions outside of your eating disorder, they also provide easy and effective ways to meet new people who share similar interests. Most of my friends while I was in school were either in the same classes as I or in the same clubs and groups. Striking up a conversation

---

Hobbies to Explore

- Knitting or crocheting
- Taking a class
- Visiting a museum
- Writing (such as fiction, poetry, or in your journal)
- Art (such as painting, drawing, or sculpting)
- Crossword puzzles
- Reading
- Playing an instrument or singing in a choir
- Traveling
- Volunteering
- Meditation

---

with a new person is much easier when you have something in common to discuss.

Spirituality

Whether or not you consider yourself to be religious, exploring spirituality can be an important part of recovery. As I worked through my eating disorder, I began to attend a local church near my apartment every week, not just for religious direction, but also for the social connection that a community of people brings. It helped me gain perspective on the importance of food in the grand scheme of the universe. Did it *really* matter what I ate for dinner?

Being interested in science and nature, I also felt a sense of calm and connection by being outside, even just sitting on my balcony in a lawn chair. When I was in treatment at a facility in the mountains, I found the change of scenery to be enormously healing. Watching the birds and squirrels playing always put a smile on my face. Adopting a cat made me understand the true importance of companionship and yarn. Having someone depend on me for care was a huge motivation to get better and stay better.

Animal Therapy (aka "Furry Prozac")

Adopting my cat from a local shelter was one of the most healing experiences of my recovery. Aria was a teen mom who was abused and abandoned after her former owners found out she was pregnant with kittens. After she had given birth, I took her in, where I spent six months coaxing her out from underneath my couch. Having a living creature that depended on me for food, water, and shelter helped me re-prioritize my values. I had to stay healthy for Aria. It also gave me a better perspective on how my parents and friends were trying to care for *me.* I would never let my cat starve or go thirsty. If she were unable to eat, I would stuff her, clawing and meowing, into her kitty carrier and drag her to the vet's. No questions asked. Except "Why don't I clip her darling little fingernails more often?"

Aria has been my major lifeline these past two years. She provides unconditional love and a potent reminder of the important things in life: naps, licks, and tuna.

Treating Yourself Properly

Recovering from an eating disorder means that you will have to nourish your mind, body, and soul. Keeping my mind sharp was a real incentive to me as I recovered, and I read hundreds of books during the process. It was amazing for me to be able to read a chapter from a book from start to finish and not think of gnawing on the pages. Or be so distracted by food that I couldn't even finish a single paragraph. As well, I wanted to feel a purpose in my life, a desire to get out of bed in the morning. I slowly expanded my life to include more friends and

Learning that I could eat what I wanted and not get fat was very reassuring.

hobbies. First, however, I had to nourish my soul with proper food so that I could be free to do everything else. Learning that I could eat what I wanted and not get fat was very reassuring. With everything I mentioned, it was important to learn how to play.

The deeper I fell into the eating disorder, the more I found myself getting stingy. Not just with food, but with everything in life. I didn't deserve to eat, I didn't deserve to spend money on myself, and I didn't deserve to have fun. I bought the cheapest of everything I could find. Even though I am on a very limited budget right now, I have learned to be extravagant in small doses, and where it will most enhance my quality of life. I buy nice coffee for myself, just because I enjoy it, and don't go out for coffee as much. I still enjoy plenty of books, but first check my local library before I drop 20 bucks on a book I'll read once. I buy overpriced unmentionables at Victoria's Secret just because they make me feel good about myself. I treat myself to high quality cheeses and breads at the specialty store every now and then. I know how to save money on things I don't care about (shoes, clothes, car stuff) so that I can treat myself to the items I truly enjoy.

Affirmations: Rewiring Your Brain

As I've said, a healthy and positive sense of self-esteem is vital to eating disorder recovery. Of course, you don't just start thinking that you're wonderful overnight. Building self-esteem is a process. In order to do so, you need to rewire your brain. And yes, you *can* try this at home. When a therapist of mine told me to do affirmations, I almost fell out of my chair laughing. I was *not* going to stand up in front of the mirror and say lovey-dovey crap to myself and believe it. No way. My therapist told me I didn't have to believe it; I just had to do it. I thought she was full of it.

I began simply, with statements like, "I am building confidence," or "I am willing to try new things." Something that was moderately believable. Every day, I said something positive to myself. It took a month or two for things to take, but eventually I did get a warm fuzzy feeling when I said these to myself. Just a little while ago, I made myself an affirmation chalkboard so I could be reminded of positive things about myself every time I walked by. Writing on the bathroom mirror in bar soap, lipstick, or dry erase marker is also fun.

Try this experiment: Move one of the garbage bins in your house. How often do you go back to the "old" spot? At first, it's probably quite a bit. Your brain *knows* to go there. You don't have to think about it. And each time you go back to the old spot, you have to reroute your brain and yourself to get to the new spot. After a while, though, you'll begin to automatically go to the new spot. It's the same with affirmations: Take out the ED garbage. You don't need it. And I know of a landfill that's just waiting for new additions.

Feelings Chase Behaviors

Affirmations, however, only do so much. There comes a time when you have to start living out your new thoughts. The catch, however, is that you usually have to start acting before you really feel like it. As mentioned, my former therapist loved to repeat the phrase "feelings chase behaviors." I had been complaining about meals, about how I wanted to wait until I wanted to eat in order to pick up the fork. "But I don't want to eat!" I protested. "This isn't fair!" She looked at me and said, "The only way to begin to want to eat and get over your fears about eating is to start eating *even though you don't want to*."

I couldn't grasp that. For a second, I thought she had grown a second head.

Seeing as I was in residential treatment, I wasn't allowed to skip meals, so I had to eat even though I didn't feel like it. The first few days were like I was a guinea pig for a new form of torture. The anxiety and fear and anger were almost unbearable (my roommate told me that although my emotions weren't unbearable, I certainly was!) Then, after a couple of months passed, I noticed a slight shift. I was eating foods almost without fear that had previously sent me spinning. In fact, I looked forward to when those foods appeared on the menu.

I still have days when my eating disorder tells me not to eat, or to binge and purge, or to overexercise. However, the only way I will ever stop feeling like engaging in the eating disorder is to behave as if I don't want to. The feelings will follow.

Adding the "And"

"I'm stupid." "I'm fat." "I'm lazy." "I'm gross." "I'm disgusting." These were all thoughts that whirred through my mind, fed to me by my eating disorder (he certainly didn't feed me anything else!). My mind would start spinning, and these thoughts would come faster and faster and faster. *I'mstupidI'mfatI'mlazy I'mgrossI'mdisgusting* . . . one right after another. I needed to slow my brain down, only I didn't know how to apply the brakes.

What I learned to do was lengthen the sentences. The negative thoughts I was having usually kept me from living life and nourishing all aspects of myself. My therapist told me that she didn't know how to change thoughts, but she did know how to change behaviors. Therefore, I needed to add the word "and" to these negative thoughts. Like, "I'm feeling fat AND I'm going to eat dinner tonight." Or, "I'm stupid AND I'm going to sign up for a new class." Feeling bad about yourself certainly makes it harder to go out and try new things, but it's no excuse for not doing them.

I put off going to treatment many times because I was afraid. I thought that if I was afraid, then I couldn't pick up the phone and make that call. I finally realized that I could feel the fear and still ask about different treatment options. My eating disorder told me that I wasn't worth the help, that I needed to lose more weight before I got help, that I was too hopeless of a case for help to even make a difference. I was scared. And I still made that call.

> *I finally realized that I could feel the fear and still ask about different treatment options.*

It was my eating disorder that didn't want me to call. Your eating disorder won't want you to, either. Just remember what *you* want to do.

Breaking the Rules

My eating disorder kept me imprisoned with a series of strict rules meant to make me feel horrible about myself. It was similar to an emotionally and physically abusive spouse: The eating disorder destroyed my self-esteem until I was too afraid to leave him. He was controlling, vain, and manipulative. But at least I had the eating disorder. Who else would ever want to be around me?

Part of recovery was breaking the rules my eating disorder had for me. Even though I still sometimes scan the menu for the low-fat items when I am out at a restaurant, I also order the entree I think I would enjoy most. If I feel I have overeaten, I still eat my next meal or snack. I no longer force myself to exercise if I am sick and tired. I sometimes treat myself to a book or item of clothing when I am out shopping, although my eating disorder tries to convince me I am not worth it.

I pierced my nose to be rebellious and celebrate my new, healthy body. Each time I do these things, I continually lessen the grip the eating disorder has on my life.

Remembering the Real You

I have baby photos of myself hanging on my wall, all manner of them, a progression of my life before the eating disorder took over. My mom gave them to me, a collage to hang up as I entered residential treatment for the last time. This baffled me: Why did I need to remember what I looked like when I was little?

Because that was who I was fighting for. The little girl who needed protection from the eating disorder. The little girl who was "enough." The little girl who I couldn't insult or degrade, despite the fact that I regularly did so to her older version. I realized that this sweet, beautiful girl didn't deserve the mistreatment that my eating disorder had heaped upon her. She had done nothing so awful that required her to starve herself, or to eat large amounts of food and force herself to throw it up. She needed to be protected.

I began to realize that I was the only person who could protect that little girl. I taped those pictures to my refrigerator, to my toilet seat, to the full-length mirror in my apartment, as a potent reminder of who I was on the inside. I knew that the little girl in the photos was me, even if I saw something hideous staring back at me from the mirror. It took me a very long time to remember that both of us were the same person, and both of us needed protection from the eating disorder. She was too young to fight; she needed me.

I still look at my baby albums with a sense of disconnect—how could that be me? How could I be smiling? How could I be eating birthday cake without fear? How could I have friends?

These were all ideas that were foreign to me at one time. At first it made me sad, to realize that this little girl would turn into me. I couldn't believe that I had a history outside of the eating disorder, and it was painful to remember that. I am still working to try and understand that I am one and the same as this precious person, and that we both deserve a life without an eating disorder.

Medical Issues in Recovery and Beyond

It can be frustrating when, even though you're very far into recovery, your life is still marked by the physical consequences of an eating disorder. The effects of starvation, even short-term starvation, can take years to reverse. If someone in China sneezes, I get a cold. Bone mass can decrease quite rapidly, especially in girls and women who have lost their periods. It did in me, and I was diagnosed with osteoporosis at 21. Any time I have vomiting or diarrhea, I worry about my potassium level falling, like it did when I was purging, so I have my potassium checked whenever I get sick.

As annoying as appointments like this can be, I remind myself that this is what I need to do in order to stay healthy, and that throwing in the towel and going back to eating disordered behaviors is only going to make things worse. What's more, my body is gradually healing itself. My bone mass is slowly improving now that I am back to a normal weight, eating sufficient amounts of both dairy products and fats and taking calcium supplements twice a day. You can't change the effects that the illness has had on you in the

You can't change the effects that the illness has had on you in the past, but with diligence you can affect your future by making healthy choices now.

past, but with diligence you can affect your future by making healthy choices now.

Food for Life

If an eating disorder isn't about food, then why do I have to eat?

I sat on a loveseat across from my dietician one afternoon and asked her this. My eating disorder really wanted to know the answer to this and was all ears.

She looked me in the eyes and said, "Whether or not your eating disorder is really 'about' food is irrelevant; if you want to get better, you still have to stop starving, binge eating, and purging." Then, she reminded me of the times when I was caught in the vicious OCD cycle of hand-washing and obsessing over germs. I could learn all number of new ways to deal with and alleviate my overwhelming anxiety, but unless I stopped washing, my life wouldn't really improve.

My dietician asked me to read a summary of a study conducted on healthy young men at the University of Minnesota in the 1940s. These men volunteered to have their daily caloric intake restricted to one-half of its usual level and then be observed for six months. During this time, the similarities between these men and people with eating disorders were striking: They became depressed, anxious, and despondent. They spent all their waking hours obsessing about food. They even occasionally binged! Only when they were allowed unlimited access to food and had returned to their natural weights did these thoughts abate.

Resuming normal eating habits is often one of the hardest parts of recovery. It is physically and mentally exhausting. I was frequently uncomfortably full, and I was uncomfortable with *being* full. Only by continuing to eat and follow the meal plan

How Otherwise Healthy People Respond to Starvation

The men who participated in the Minnesota Starvation Study experienced a number of personality and behavioral changes as their calories were cut and they began to lose weight. As time went on, they began to:

- Experience depression and emotional distress
- Find themselves preoccupied with food and cooking
- Hide food to consume in secret
- Increase their physical activity to receive more food
- Attempt to fill themselves up with water, coffee, tea, and gum
- Lose interest in normal life activities
- Lose their sense of humor

In order to regain their lost weight, these men found they had to consume large amounts of food. Even though they ate many times their typical, pre-study intake, they remained hungry as their bodies began to recover. It took up to a year for their hunger and fullness cues to re-regulate.

Remembering the results of this study really helped me understand that the emotional changes I was experiencing as part of the eating disorder were partly physiological and would lessen as I began to eat.

provided by my dietician did these feelings begin to change. A good friend and fellow young woman in recovery from anorexia reminded me that food was my medicine. However, just like chemotherapy for cancer patients, it could make you feel, well, awful sometimes. My digestive system had essentially forgotten how to work properly. The anxiety created by weight restoration, and even just eating normal meals, nearly drove me out of my mind. However, just like a cancer patient knows that chemotherapy will help them in the long

... even with all of the nasty side effects, I knew that continuing to eat was my ticket to recovery.

run, even with all of the nasty side effects, I knew that continuing to eat was my ticket to recovery.

Recovery at All Costs

After hitting a really low point in my eating disorder, I vowed to recover at all costs. Whatever it took, I would do it. If that meant trying a new, scary food, then I would do it. If it meant moving to a cheaper apartment closer to work so that I could pay for food and therapy, then I would do it. It meant that oversleeping was no excuse for not eating, and that I had to put groceries higher up on my budget than books. It meant always carrying a snack in my purse so that I had no excuse not to eat. It meant taking a lower stress, lower paying job so that I could be closer to my treatment team and have more energy to put into recovery.

It means that now, I never trip over my bathroom scale because I gleefully threw it in a dumpster on garbage day. Now, my fridge contains a wide variety of foods and leftovers. I actually use my cookbooks to prepare recipes rather than just slobbering over them. My kitchen table is often filled with food and people. I am not afraid to miss a workout to meet a friend for coffee to cheer her up after a rough day.

How far are *you* willing to go?

Chapter Six

Dealing With the World
While in Recovery

By now you're probably thinking, "Great. So now what? I know how and why to seek treatment, how to get my family and friends to help me, and how to treat myself right when in recovery. But what comes next? What happens when I have to go to school, or work, or when I move away to college?" Hell if I know. I don't have a recipe book for this. There is no one right way. What I can offer is advice, and ways of coping throughout recovery that have helped me.

Whereas the previous chapter focused on how to meet the emotional and mental challenges of your own personal recovery, this chapter offers some simple, everyday tactics that will help you deal with school, family, work—in other words, the outside world—while recovering from an eating disorder. Let's face it—dealing with people and responsibilities can be difficult even under the best of circumstances. The following are strategies that helped me get through each day of work, school, and everything in between during my long fight against the eating disorder, and which may also help you to keep your recovery on track and to stay healthy.

Talking to Family and Friends About Your Eating Disorder

While I never had to tell most of my family and friends that I had an eating disorder (they were the ones that, for months and months, were telling *me* that I had a problem), I eventually had to confess that they were right and that I could not get through this alone. All I could hear were the "I told you so's" that I imagined my parents uttering. Thankfully, they never did. They simply nodded in acceptance and began to mobilize resources. Not everyone is this lucky—sometimes parents may throw their hands up in despair, and you will have to find help from friends, school counselors, clergy, or other important people in your life. Many times, people who care about you are willing to help; they may blunder some at first, but as long as they are willing to educate themselves, then you are off to a good start.

The best way to open the lines of communication about your eating disorder is to approach your parents when they have plenty of time to discuss the issue. Use "I" statements to describe your experience ("I feel fat when I eat") rather than "you" statements ("You make fattening food"). If you can create an environment of open and honest communication emanating from yourself, it will probably make it easier for your family and friends to be open and honest as well.

Be prepared for a variety of responses, ranging from support to tears, denial to rage, and everything in between. Keep in mind that a strong reaction doesn't indicate that this person doesn't care about you and your situation. It just means that he or she is worried or scared or angry for not notic-

Keep in mind that a strong reaction doesn't indicate that this person doesn't care about you and your situation.

ing it sooner. Often people will have been aware that something was unusual about your behavior, and will be glad to finally know what is going on. Unfortunately, there is still intense stigma around mental health issues in general, as well as a general misunderstanding about eating disorders in particular, which may make it more difficult for a loved one to accept that you are suffering from a mental illness. Educational pamphlets, and information printed off of reputable Web sites (see the Resources section of this book) can be helpful should this be the case. Lastly, you might lend them this book if you feel it will help them understand what you are going through.

Enlisting Support During Recovery

When my parents began to insist that I had an eating disorder, I was reluctant to begin treatment because I thought I could "do it on my own." Unfortunately, even though it seemed like I had thought my way into the eating disorder, I couldn't think myself out of it. Both professional and personal support was needed. I have never met anyone who successfully recovered from an eating disorder without outside help. We need either professional support, or the support of friends and family.

. . . no one can support you if they don't know what's wrong.

When appropriate, it's helpful to involve your immediate family in your recovery. Not all families are willing and able to assist during this process, but many parents and siblings do want to help. One of the best ways of enlisting their support is to be open about your eating disorder and the resulting struggles. I've learned the hard way that no one can support you if they don't know what's wrong. Your family can't read minds.

They won't know how to help unless you tell them. I've found that a lot of education and family therapy (see Chapter 4) can be really useful in facilitating this dialogue. My parents are much better now at knowing that "I feel fat!" is much more about how I'm feeling emotionally than about the size of my butt. They know that times of stress are when I need the most support. They know where healthy support ends and interference begins.

It's also important to involve your friends in your recovery. My friends know when Starbucks therapy is appropriate, or when it's time to stay in and watch a movie. However, they only know this because I have told them. It took many therapy sessions and years of practice before I acquired even marginal finesse and ease in successfully asking for their help. It then took even longer to accept that not everyone had equal abilities to support me. Don't ask for bananas from someone who doesn't have bananas (or so says my therapist).

Being open about your eating disorder with people outside of your immediate circle of family and friends (and even within that circle) is a matter of personal preference. Sometimes, it can help decrease the shame that can surround eating disordered behaviors, as well as provide other avenues of support. On the other hand, knowing that you have a mental illness can bias people against you, especially colleges and potential employers. So telling people doesn't mean that you wear a sandwich board screaming "I have an eating disorder!" in bright red letters. Discretion is advised in determining who to tell. Talking to your parents and friends about how open you want to be can help prevent misunderstandings. Outright lying about your illness can be problematic, and there are plenty of other ways to prevent unwanted discussions about your condition.

Dealing With Dumb Comments, Part I

It's almost a given that you will get dumb comments from people. They may remark upon any changes in personal habits or body weight and shape as a result of your eating disorder, and their comments can range from simple curiosity to pure boneheaded stupidity. While most people really do mean well when they ask questions, they're usually not very well informed, so they frequently have the opposite effect. I've received numerous idiotic comments from people who don't have a clue about eating disorders. Highlights include:

- *I wish I had an eating disorder, too!*
- *So, do you just, like, not eat or something?*
- *Can you teach me how to lose weight so well?*
- *Do you eat your cake and puke it too?*
- *Do you have AIDS?*
- *Just eat already!*
- *If you don't give up your eating disorder, you're going to hell.*

I've found these comments to be a great opportunity for both a) sarcasm and b) a little education about eating disorders. The comment that provides the best opportunity (and the greatest ire on my part) is when people say they wish they could have a little case of anorexia. Oh, really? So you want to have osteoporosis at the age of 23? Permanently messed up intestines from laxative abuse? A depleted college fund? You want to skip communion at church because you're afraid of the calories in the bread and communion wine? Pass up going to your friend's bridal shower because you can't miss your workout? Still want anorexia? When people tell me I'm hearing the voice of Satan and that I need to repent, I say that the worst version of hell has to be better than this.

Sometimes brutal honesty like this is the best way to deal with those comments. I've found most people leave you alone after that. Of course, I don't recommend you tell people how to lose weight, but telling them that an eating disorder is not the way to go is pretty effective. It's important to remember that these statements are less about you than they are about that person's perceptions about him or herself. In the end, it's up to you to determine how open you want to be about your eating disorder. With some people, evasion is the way to go because they cannot be trusted to keep what you have to say in confidence.

In the end, it's up to you to determine how open you want to be about your eating disorder.

Everyday Life: The 23 Hours Each Day When You're Not in Therapy

Therapy is extremely useful and will likely be a large support for you during recovery, as will be family and friends. The point of all this therapy and hard work isn't to learn how people can catch you when you fall; it's to learn how to land on your own two feet. There are some aspects of life in recovery that can be managed with the help of family and friends, while other changes must be carried out by you alone. While you will likely have to alter some of the strategies below to fit your individual needs, they are intended to give you general hints and a starting point.

Life in Middle School and High School

Dealing with school during recovery can be extremely difficult and anxiety-provoking. The best bet is to have a plan for how you will deal with teachers, schoolwork, and other classmates. Especially when dealing with teachers, it is usually most effective to enlist the aid of your parents and treatment team to provide written proof of any exceptions you might need. Most teachers are very willing to accommodate your needs, ranging from giving alternative exams or providing more time for tests, to easing up a homework load, to allowing you to work with a tutor for home schooling. This can be useful when frequent therapist and doctor appointments cause you to miss classes on a regular basis. I used these methods when I got sick with severe bronchitis and frequently couldn't make it to my first hour class during my junior year of high school. It really aided in my recovery by letting my body get the rest it needed.

Dealing With Classmates

Classmates, on the other hand, can be much trickier. Middle school and high school are known for cliques, which can be a source of gossip and other rumors. These can't always be prevented, and there is a fine line between being open enough to prevent rumors and protecting your own privacy. Many people simply want to know out of concern and curiosity, though it can be different ratios of each. Especially in the lunchroom, it can be difficult to eat responsibly when friends are on diets and talking about food and weight. It's best to insist on changing the subject. You don't always have to say why, but you have the right to speak up about such issues.

Life in College and Beyond

College is a time when eating disorders can flourish, due to the increased stress and decreased structure and supervision. After a brief bout of anorexia as a preteen, my eating disorder began in earnest in college, starting slowly during my freshman year and building steam throughout my sophomore year. By the beginning of my senior year, I was so exhausted that I had no choice but to take a semester off to enter residential treatment. Considering that I was a top student at my school, this reality was devastating. My whole existence outside of the eating disorder was centered on school. Without that, I was lost. The semester off, however, proved lifesaving. With my workload, I never would have had the energy to devote myself fully to recovery.

The decision to take a semester or year off of college is a very personal one. I know plenty of people who recovered while remaining full-time students. I also know plenty of people who needed that time off to regroup and work more intensively toward recovery. Having applied to graduate school, I know that most schools (and most employers) look most closely at what courses you have taken. Taking a semester off is a fairly common occurrence, and so it tends not to be questioned closely. Talk to your treatment team about this, and they can provide you with some guidance.

As with middle and high school, talking to your college professors and other instructors about your issues may allow you to alter your workload to maximize your recovery should you choose to stay in school. You don't have to disclose the exact reason you need alterations; simply saying that you have a medical condition typically provides as much information as an instructor requires. If you have particularly supportive professors, it might be helpful to tell them about your eating disorder, since they could be a good source of support.

Many college administrations are now beginning to realize the impact of eating disorders upon the student population, and have on-campus support groups, as well as free psychological and nutritional counseling. I received a semester of free weekly counseling from my school, and many people have done the same. This is especially convenient if you are no longer covered by your parents' insurance plans. Even if you are not in college, the campus counseling centers can provide community referrals.

Many college administrations are now beginning to realize the impact of eating disorders upon the student population, and have on-campus support groups...

Another aspect to grappling with an eating disorder during college is the sense of isolation that it brings. Between my eating disorder behaviors and schoolwork, I had essentially no time for friends or socializing. All of that was done at my part-time on-campus job at the school newspaper. Even then, it was difficult when the staff would go out for dinner or drinks and I was too afraid to join in. Relieving that isolation was a monumental task. What helped me was staying involved in organizations where I found social support, attending religious services on a regular basis, and reducing the total number of classes I took each semester to leave me with more energy and time to build meaningful friendships and relationships.

Life on the Job

Combined with school, as well as therapy and dietician appointments, an after-school job or internship requires a careful juggling act. From personal experience, I have found recovery work to be so difficult that I needed to de-stress my life as much as possible, so I didn't have a job. On the other hand, when I was away from college, going to a part-time job for ten hours a week got me out of the house and provided a distraction from the eating disorder thinking.

Get a feeling about your supervisor and whether or not you would feel safe telling him or her about your eating disorder. If you decide not to, you can just say that you have a medical problem that needs close monitoring. Your supervisor need not know any more than that—your eating disorder is a personal matter, and you can choose how much information you disclose. However, make sure your supervisor knows of your need for meal and other breaks so that you don't become too hungry. Again, you can just say that you have to eat frequently because of a medical condition. All of my supervisors, even in high-pressure jobs, have been extremely accommodating and supportive of me, even allowing me to shift around my schedule for meals and appointments.

Walking the Walk and Talking the Talk

When I was deep in the throes of anorexia, I thought that once I ate a few slices of pie, I would be "cured," could leave the hospital, and go back to my daily life. Let's just say that if my miracle apple pie cure had worked, I would be rich by now. Recovery consists of both physical and mental rehabilitation. For most people, the physical recovery tends to occur before the psychological symptoms abate. This creates a strange disconnect where you might look better as your body heals, yet the eating disordered thoughts are still very intense. *Eating properly and/or maintaining a healthy weight are NOT the sole indicators of recovery.* Other essential indicators include a decrease in obsessive thoughts, an ability to eat and digest food without fear, a decrease in body image distortion, and a return to normal daily life.

After I was first diagnosed with an eating disorder, I read any number of books and Web sites on recovery, hoping I could magically "cure" myself. I thought the magic key was somewhere out there, and if I looked hard enough, I would find it. The key was out there, though, and I had probably even found it on several occasions. Problem was, I never thought of actually putting the key in the lock and turning it. Advice is only good when you put it into action. You don't have to do everything I suggest, but you do have to take action and pursue your recovery aggressively. You may falter from

... once you commit to recovering and staying healthy, the specter of the eating disorder will decrease while the quality of your life will greatly improve.

time to time—a subject I'll discuss in the next chapter—but once you commit to recovering and staying healthy, the specter of the eating disorder will decrease while the quality of your life will greatly improve.

Chapter Seven

Relapse: There and Back Again

A h, relapse. That dreaded word—especially in treatment centers. Relapse is defined as the resurgence of eating-disorder symptoms or the deterioration of a person's condition following an initially successful response to treatment. Relapse is common among those with eating disorders, though it is unclear how common because of inconsistent ideas about what exactly constitutes a relapse. One study of 95 patients between the ages of 12 and 18 estimated that up to 30% re-lapsed back into anorexia following discharge from an inpatient treatment center. Relapse rates for bulimia are thought to be similar.

While relapse may be common, it is not inevitable, nor does it mean that you can never truly recover. A relapse is a chance to learn from what got you into that tough spot—*after you have gotten back on track*. If you come upon a car accident on a deserted road, you don't stop to ask if someone was drunk, was not paying attention, or could not see. You get out of your car to help the passengers. Then, the police can come back and analyze the scene.

A relapse is a chance to learn…

It's the same idea with a relapse. First get the passengers out and to the hospital. Then analyze the scene. The analysis will provide lots of information that can be used to make changes to the road, or to laws about drinking and driving.

On my own road to recovery, I made many wrong turns. I would conquer one particular eating disorder behavior only to substitute it with another. Sometimes, the same behaviors would return with an astounding vengeance that frightened me. I repeatedly struggled and fell, got back up, moved forward, moved backward, and even just sat still for quite a while. However, as one of my friends says, "As long as you keep putting

Signs of Relapse

- Increase in obsessive thinking about food and weight
- Wanting to be in control all the time
- Perfectionistic attitudes
- Wanting to escape from stressful situations
- Feeling hopeless about work, relationships or life
- Believing you will be happy and successful if thin
- Feelings of being "too fat," even though people say otherwise
- Wanting to isolate
- Being unable to use your support systems
- Being dishonest with those helping you about your symptoms
- Looking in the mirror often
- Daily weighing
- Avoiding certain foods because of the calorie content
- Purchasing mostly diet foods
- Skipping meals
- Excessive exercising
- Wearing only loose-fitting clothes
- Thoughts of suicide
- Feeling disgusted with oneself after eating

(Excerpted from *The Body Betrayed: A Deeper Understanding of Women, Eating Disorders, and Treatment,* by Katherine Zerbe.)

> I do believe in full recovery, but I also know that I cannot ever forget that I suffered from an eating disorder,...

one foot in front of the other, you'll eventually get somewhere."

Even as I write this book, I am still in recovery from my eating disorder. I'm not perfect. Although I am at a healthy weight, I still have days when I look into the mirror and cringe. There are still times when I think I can lose "just a few pounds" and stop when I want. The difference is that I now know the dangers of going back to the eating disorder. I do believe in full recovery, but I also know that I cannot ever forget that I suffered from an eating disorder, lest I return to my destructive behaviors. I made that mistake before, during my own struggle with relapse, and I cannot afford to make it again.

One Step Forward, Two Steps Back

In the six months after I was released from my last trip to the psychiatric ward for anorexia, I clung to life, barely hanging on by my fingernails. Life was very new, and very raw. I graduated from college with a degree in biochemistry and math, but lacked a job. Out of desperation, I accepted the first offer that came along, a research position in a genetics lab at a major research hospital. It was miserable. I was bored out of my skull. I love numbers and computers, but managing a database and running DNA tests didn't occupy my mind as much as I needed. I was also living alone for the first time in my life.

All of these changes, all at once, did not bode well for me.

My brain, seeking to find something to do all day, began once again to obsess over food. With the major concerns of finishing my college thesis out of the way, the eating disorder voice roared back to life. Since I soon learned the routines of the research lab, my mind seized upon food and weight to chew upon. Without the support and structure of home, I found myself floundering. I did not know how to fight the eating disorder. All of my treatment before had focused on the more immediate needs of medical and psychiatric stabilization, and I had yet to learn how to fully break free from anorexia.

The crap really hit the fan when yet another medical problem materialized: I had one seizure, then another, although I was ED behavior–free in both instances. My doctors couldn't really figure out why the seizures were occurring and threw around a number of the standard causes of epilepsy, but one stood out in my mind, echoing back and forth. *Brain damage.* Seizures can be caused by brain damage. Could starvation have caused brain damage? I reeled in shock. It is known that some metabolic aberrations, like low levels of sodium in the bloodstream, can cause seizures when people are starving. But, could I have experienced *long-term* effects that led to epilepsy? I couldn't stop worrying that I had permanently damaged my body. I didn't think this would happen to me. The consequences were worse: no driver's license for over six months. You can take the girl out of Starbucks, but you can't take the need for Starbucks out of the girl. This had to have been the biggest blow: being completely dependent on other people for such basic necessities as *coffee.*

While the anti-seizure medications I began taking were successful at controlling my seizures, they also caused extensive weight gain. I was unaware of this, and began to freak out as I routinely ate my way through my kitchen cupboards. I blamed it on moral weakness and yearned for the feelings of self-control that accompanied anorexia. As time passed, I grew so frantic about my increased food intake that I began to purge, which quickly turned into a two-year long relapse into a binge-purge-restrict cycle that never seemed to end. It never occurred to me that the restricting following a binge and purge only perpetuated the cycle.

Throughout this time, I had finished up my job in the research lab and begun a master's program at the University of Michigan. I enjoyed my classes tremendously, even though they involved extremely challenging work. The amount of work, however, only fueled the binge-purge-restrict cycle even more. All day, I prayed that I would "stay strong" and not binge that night. The few times that I didn't binge promoted the belief that one day, I would stop binge eating. I stayed honest with my dietician during this time, believing that she could help me out of this predicament. I waited for things to "click." Problem is, things never click until you start doing the work.

> *All day, I prayed that I would "stay strong" and not binge that night.*

The irony is that I stopped binge eating and purging because of a crush on a guy. He was the oral surgeon who removed my wisdom teeth. Because I had become violently ill previously on strong painkillers, he gave me a prescription for extra-strength Advil. He explained that vomiting could cause the stitches to come out and create a dry socket. I didn't know quite what that was, but it sounded painful. And I didn't want to return and admit why my stitches had come out. So I stopped throwing up. Cold turkey. After white-knuckling my way through the first few weeks, I found fewer and fewer urges to purge as time went on.

My weight stabilized at that point. Mentally and physically, I felt better than I had in years, even though my thinking remained quite obsessed with food and weight. I still thought I was too fat and I vowed that one day, I would lose the excess weight from the medications.

Return to Anorexia

My slide back into anorexia began so slowly that I did not recognize this relapse for what it was. Each step was so small, I could write it off. I never realized I was on dangerous ground until it was too late. My second year of graduate school was stressful beyond words. I often spent 12 hours a day in the computer lab finishing assignments and projects. My brother was getting married in November, and I was one of the bridesmaids (complete with the skimpy dress and dyed-to-match shoes). My first book was scheduled to be published. And I simply cracked.

I stayed in school by the skin of my teeth. I dropped a class to ease up the workload, and found myself really enjoying the electives I got to take during my last semester of grad school. I managed to rally for a while. Unfortunately, I began to rely on a temporary solution to carry me through permanently. As I completed researching and writing my thesis, and began to apply for a job, the stress and uncertainty over employment once again overwhelmed me. My weight and vitals continued on their downward slide, but just as I was considering more intensive treatment, I was hired by the Michigan Health Department in an exciting but high-stress position. I failed to put my recovery first, and I had no idea how quickly I would be required to face the consequences.

The long hours, constant stress and resurging eating disorder symptoms wore me out. Suddenly, eating became less of a concern as sleeping took priority. I collapsed as soon as I got home from work and didn't wake up until the next morning.

The depression also returned and I decided to try a new anti-depressant in order to help.

Starting on the new antidepressant was the breaking point for me. I had been teetering on the edge of more intensive treatment for over a year, and as I started eating less, the anorexia, tenuously held at bay for so long, resumed its death grip on my brain. At first, I zoomed with energy, not even feeling the need to eat. Surely I didn't need something as banal as *food*. I stopped sleeping normally, tossing and turning all night. To funnel my excess energy, I began to walk around my apartment complex for hours at a time and did my chores at a frenetic pace I couldn't understand. I didn't know then that the antidepressant had sent me spinning into an episode of hypomania, almost identical to the one that had occurred four and a half years previous.

A spectacular high, however, is always followed by a spectacular low. Just like Newton's Second Law of Motion—what goes up must come down—I crashed within a week. I returned to the doctor's office with excessive fatigue and was finally diagnosed with mononucleosis, to which my weight loss (noticeable, but not excessive) was attributed. I had a follow-up appointment the next week.

As the first hunger pangs emerged, I ignored them. I did not want to feel them, no longer knew what hunger *meant*, and was too exhausted to do anything about it. I assembled every excuse in the book to refrain from eating: I was too stressed, too busy, too unsure about the proper foods to eat. So I whittled my diet down from an already narrow list, and continued to exercise as much as I could. I hauled out my dusty old bathroom scale from under the bed, and proceeded to call upon it as judge and jury every time I set foot into my miniature bathroom. As astonished as I was at how much weight had fallen off my naturally thin frame, a nasty voice in the base of my skull hissed,

"Lose more! You're still too fat! You have NO self-control!" What could I say? I turned to all manner of pills that I thought might aid weight loss. I became phobic of nearly everything I put into my mouth. I systematically denied myself all of the necessities of life: sleep, food, and water. No rationality can explain this. I was not vain, or seeking attention. Instead, I was embarrassed and ashamed of my behavior.

The next several weeks passed in a gray haze. I returned to the doctor and was gently questioned about my weight loss. I pleaded stress and fatigue. "I'll make an effort to eat more. Really I will." By the next week, my weight and vital signs had dropped so dramatically, my doctor's gentle concern turned into stark worry. I returned the third week with virtually no blood pressure and slow, weak pulse. An EKG was ordered and turned up abnormalities. I vowed to go to the urgent care clinic attached to the local hospital for tests after I had seen my therapist. I walked in her door and was immediately driven to the emergency room. Low potassium was found, as well as ketones in my urine—signs of a starving body. They ordered me to drink some juice, eat some graham crackers, and take potassium supplements. The doctor was confused as to my signs and symptoms, and so told me to "watch out and be careful." My mother drove me back to my apartment and, right before flipping off the light to go to bed, I took more pills. I had simply lost my mind.

I continued working at the state health department until a follow-up appointment the next week. I was once again told I needed IV fluids. I allowed myself to be rehydrated in the emergency room, constantly fighting the urge to rip out the needle and make a run for it. Time sped up and, five days later, I found myself flying across the country to a residential treatment center, where I spent the next seven months.

Back in Residential Treatment

I fought the system with all of my energy. I cried through many meals. When I couldn't finish, a staff member would sit with me at the table until I had eaten my meal. However, as time passed and my body and mind regained strength, I found the food less threatening and began to open up to my therapists and to the other residents during group therapy. Various medical problems cropped up along the way, delaying the process of weight restoration. By the end of my time in treatment, I was strong enough mentally and physically to leave when the time was right.

My journey isn't over now that I am out of treatment and back into my real life. I still struggle daily, but now I have the skills I need to keep eating and reach out to others—one of those skills is recognizing that there *will* be setbacks from time to time. What's important to recognize is that this doesn't mean a full recovery will never be within your grasp.

Relapse Prevention

Though it is impossible to predict for sure who will relapse and who will not, or when a relapse might take place, researchers have pinpointed some factors that seem to protect against relapse. For example, one study of adults with eating disorders indicated that if the weight gained during hospitalization is maintained for a year after discharge, the risk of relapse declines significantly. In other words, the longer you can maintain a normal weight after being in the hospital, the lower your risk is of relapsing—so it's especially important for you to focus on recovery in the first few months following discharge.

...the longer you can maintain a normal weight after being in the hospital, the lower your risk is of relapsing...

The same psychological treatments that I described in Chapter 4 are also used to prevent relapse. Cognitive-behavior therapy and the Maudsley method have been shown to be particularly effective in preventing a resurgence of symptoms. So even if you feel you've recovered fully from your eating disorder, it may be a good idea to continue with some form of long-term psychotherapy.

Though medications are not believed to be effective in underweight people with anorexia, they have been shown to be effective for those suffering from bulimia. Many mental health professionals believe that those recovering from bulimia are less likely to relapse if they continue psychopharmacological treatment for at least six months.

At the end of the day, preemptive action is the key. If you feel yourself slipping back into unhealthy eating behaviors, tell someone immediately—your parents, your doctor, or another member of your treatment team. Relapses can often be even more severe than the initial occurrence of the eating disorder, so the faster you can stop the resurgence of symptoms the better your chances are of avoiding a full-blown relapse.

The phrase I always hated hearing while new into recovery was "Isn't your life so much *better* now?" Uh, no. In some ways, it felt worse. The anxiety was worse, the physical discomfort was worse. I almost idealized the good ol' days of anorexia and bulimia, forgetting how awful I really felt back then, the life almost devoid of any sort of pleasure. However, although both recovery and an eating disorder can be hell, recovery has something positive at the end. An eating disorder only has a coffin.

The Recovery Bike

It took me two years of practice before I ever took the training wheels off of my first bike. I remember it clearly: a purple Huffy with streamers and a little plastic basket with tacky pink flowers in front. It was the summer I turned seven, and I finally got going down the road. I turned around to give my mom the thumbs-up sign, and promptly drove straight into a mailbox. After blotting off my scraped chin and elbow, I hopped right back on, and went right on riding. I had plenty of other mishaps, including wiping out on a gravel road, but I learned from each of those experiences (like, "watch where you're going" and, "don't jackknife on a dirt road"). To this day, I love the feeling of flying down a sidewalk or dirt trail.

Recovery works the same way. You try, you fall. You go back to your training wheels. You take them off again. You fall. You climb back on. You get going. You fall. You climb back on. The other most important thing to remember when riding your recovery bike is that just because you fall doesn't mean that you can't get back on and try again. Recovery from an eating disorder is difficult and it takes practice. Allow yourself to take a spill once in a while, without giving up entirely.

Allow yourself to take a spill once in a while, without giving up entirely.

Dealing with Dumb Comments, Part II

It would be nice, of course, if people stopped saying dumb things once you started recovery. Unfortunately, the comments can occasionally be even more ridiculous. Such as:

- *You look SO healthy now!*
- *So, are you going to go puke now?*
- *They fattened you up real nice.*
- *You don't LOOK like you were ever anorexic.*

Again, sometimes the best tactic is to simply walk away, especially if you don't want to discuss your eating disorder with that person. With other people, it might be useful to tell them how you interpreted their comment. If someone says you look healthier, you can feel free to say that your eating disorder tells you that healthy means you're fat, and to please not say those things. Even if the other person doesn't quite understand how your thinking works, the object is to get them to stop saying harmful things.

Then again, humor is also useful. I was told by a friendly but not-so-helpful store clerk that I looked like I was "gaining weight quite nicely." I said, "Thanks. So do you." I almost would have sold my soul to capture the expression on her face. Before walking out the door, I said, "If you keep your thoughts on my weight to yourself, I'll keep my mouth shut, too." She never said another word about my weight again.

Chapter Eight

Closure

I have written this book as a young woman in recovery from anorexia and bulimia. It has taken hundreds of thousands of dollars and hundreds and thousands of hours of hard work to get to the place in which I currently live. I get daunted, still, when I look at the road ahead of me and realize that I still have work to do. Yet I look back over the landscape I have traveled and realize how much progress I have made since I began my recovery.

For many years I wanted to recover, I just wasn't willing to put in the work involved. I wanted recovery on *my* terms: no gaining weight, no stopping binge eating and purging, no eating of fear foods. But, hey! I wanted to get better. While this was definitely something, it wasn't until I committed to full recovery and whatever that took that I started to make real progress against the eating disorder. Everyone's path to recovery takes a different route and a different amount of time; it's not a competition, it's not a race. There isn't a "perfect recovery." You will fall on your butt. You will get lost. This is okay—it's how you learn.

Author Jenni Schaefer has expressed to me her three rules of recovery from an eating disorder:

1. Your eating disorder is not an option.
2. You do whatever it takes in order to recover.
3. Never, never, never give up. Not ever.

The statistics on recovery from anorexia and bulimia are not always cheerful. However, as someone who has a degree in epidemiology and statistics, I know that a statistic says something about a *group* of people, not an individual person. You have a 100% chance of getting better if you put as much work and energy into recovery as you do into the eating disorder.

You have a 100% chance of getting better if you put as much work and energy into recovery as you do into the eating disorder.

An eating disorder didn't happen to you overnight, and it won't get better overnight. I had to sit down to fear foods and wait out urges to binge and purge many times before the fears started to lessen. Every time I thought I couldn't handle the fear and anxiety and went back to ED behaviors, I had to do a lot of backtracking to get back on course. It can be done, of course, and I'm living proof of that. As Yoda from *Star Wars* says, "Do or do not. There is no try."

Recovery always seemed like a distinct destination to me, a Disney World of sorts. The only resemblance that this idea had to the process of recovery was the presence of roller coasters. I had so many ups and downs that I became nauseated. One minute, I felt happy and hopeful, and the next I was miserable and pessimistic. I switched moods at the drop of a hat. When I was feeling down, I would frequently throw in the towel and run back to my eating disorder, arms outstretched. As time went on, I realized that the bad times wouldn't last. I never had the fear that I would be happy forever. Why would sadness be any different?

Many times, I thought that even though full recovery was possible, I couldn't recover. Not me. Sometimes, I thought I wasn't sick enough to "merit" recovery. Other times, I thought I had been too sick for too long to actually get better. Wherever you're at in your eating disorder, for however long you have been sick, full recovery *is* possible. Much of my work hinged on that belief: I had the potential to recover. Maybe not right at that moment, but, one day, I would be free of eating disordered thoughts and behaviors.

Now that my life is no longer consumed by my eating disorder, I have the time and energy to pursue the activities I love. I can write better and more clearly than when my brain was starving. I can use my experiences in overcoming anorexia and bulimia to help others, educate them on the subject, and advocate for better research, care, and insurance coverage of eating disorders. I can snuggle with my kitty and not feel guilty. I can sample desserts in a store and just relax and enjoy them.

...my worst days now are still better than my best days of anorexia and bulimia, and I have a lot more hope for the future.

Life in recovery and life after recovery will never be perfect. I desperately wish they could be, and that all of the time and energy we pour into healing would mean a one-way ticket to Utopia. That has yet to happen—though I'll let you know if it does. Yet my worst days now are still better than my best days of anorexia and bulimia, and I have a lot more hope for the future. That's something to remember as you embark upon your own journey to recovery. It can be a long, difficult road, and things may get worse before they get better, but if you commit to recovery, they will get better.

I'm not there yet, but I keep the faith. I push on.

Trials never end, of course. Unhappiness and misfortune are bound to occur as long as people live, but there is a feeling now that wasn't here before, and is not just on the surface of things, that says: We've won it. It's going to get better now. You can sort of tell these things.

—Robert M. Pirsig, *Zen and the Art of Motorcycle Maintenance*

For Caregivers of Young People With Eating Disorders

A lthough I have had years of experience in directly coping with an eating disorder, I have not been the one to cope with the person suffering from an eating disorder. My mom says that "hell" is an understatement of what life was like. It is not easy for anyone involved. The fact that you are even reading this book should be applauded. Some parents would deny their child's illness to the end of their days, while others can be so overwhelmed that they don't even know where to start.

First, let me say this: Your child's eating disorder is not your fault. It isn't. You had no control over whether or not your child got sick. Unfortunately, at this point you know that your child is sick, and so it's a matter of deciding where to go from here. Spending time on the guilt and blame game isn't going to help your child, either with yourself or with professionals. Everyone feels this guilt, the constant rumination of "What did I do that made my child sick?"

Let me repeat myself: This is *not* your fault. You didn't cause it and you can't cure it. But you can help.

What I Wish My Parents Had Known

Much of the wisdom in the eating disorder world comes from (very) hard-earned experience. So does the information in this section. Hopefully, my insights and those provided by my parents will help make your journey just a little bit easier.

Rule #1: Trust Your Instincts

If you think something is wrong, it usually is. Maybe it's not an eating disorder. But maybe it is, and studies have shown that the sooner treatment is begun, the better the outcome. Take your child to the pediatrician for a check-up. The worst that happens is that you have a perfectly healthy, if somewhat annoyed, child. Be open and honest with both your child and the pediatrician about what you suspect. Have the pediatrician check your child's growth charts and weight history. In a growing child, no amount of weight loss is healthy unless it's doctor-supervised.

Rule #2: Beware the Young Dieter

Having been a teenager and college student until fairly recently, I know all too well how common dieting and body image obsessions are. In many people, these obsessions are painful and distracting, but not life threatening. However, if your family has a history of anxiety, mood, and/or eating disorders, the stakes for starting an innocent-seeming diet can be much, much higher. Because eating disorders tend to cluster with these other mental illnesses, your child can be set up for an eating disorder without even knowing it.

Rule #3: Advocate for Your Child

Especially if your child is very young, you will need to take charge of the treatment and make sure he or she receives the help required. Denial is a common feature of eating disorders, and even adult sufferers find it almost impossible to seek help of their own volition. Especially if your child is under 18, you have the right and obligation to look after his or her psychiatric and medical health. Research all of the options. Include yourself as part of the treatment team if at all feasible—you are the person who spends the most time with your child, and the input you can supply to treatment providers is often invaluable.

Rule #4: The Eating Disorder Hates You, Your Child Does Not

I'll somewhat sheepishly admit that I've lashed out at my mother before in the midst of the eating disorder. I was confused. I was scared. I was frustrated. The emotions were so intense that I couldn't articulate them properly and simply let loose at the closest person. Part of the reason I ended up getting angry at my parents and close friends was that they were the biggest threat to the eating disorder, and therefore provoked the strongest reactions. If your child appears angry with you, especially if you are supervising meals, then it could be a positive sign because you are threatening the eating disorder.

Rule #5: Your Child Has an Illness

If your adolescent has an eating disorder, she will very likely lie to you. Your child is not lying to irritate you or because it is fun. Your child is lying because she is afraid, afraid of eating. There is also considerable shame surrounding binge eating and purging, which can lead to lying and concealing behaviors and their evidence. While it's healthy to establish honesty from everyone, whether they have an eating disorder or not, try to think of the lying as a symptom of the disease. That's not to say that lying is okay, just that eating disorders don't particularly lend themselves well to honesty. Be firm. Be supportive.

Rule #6: If Necessary, Search Until You Find a Doctor That Helps You

I may sound a little blunt here, but some doctors wouldn't recognize an eating disorder even if they were told outright what was going on. Lab tests and blood work frequently come back normal even in seriously ill people, so don't let a doctor dismiss your concerns. Find another doctor. There is one out there who will listen to you. This is especially true if you are in a population that is not traditionally believed to have people who suffer from eating disorders (i.e., if your child is not young, female, or white). Sometimes a diagnosis can take persistence, considering the high levels of denial common in both anorexia and bulimia.

Rule #7: Your Insurance Company May Not Help You—but Be Persistent

Eating disorders are considered by insurance companies to be mental illnesses, even though the physical consequences of starving, binge eating, and purging are all very real. Therefore, it can be difficult to get coverage for your child unless he or she is medically compromised. It's said that if you appeal the insurance company's decision for long enough, you will win three out of four times. I know of parents who have taken out second mortgages on their homes in order to get care for their children. There are also treatment options like the Maudsley method that allow you to re-feed your child at home without hospital care.

Rule #8: Your Kid Is Still in There

Really. I promise. Love them. Help them fight. They will return. Without an exorcist needed.

Things Not to Say to a Person Suffering From an Eating Disorder

My mom always joked that there was only one way I would interpret her comments: the exact way they *weren't* intended. My eating disorder twisted every comment and compliment to mean I was fat. Joking with her now, I say that I should have read her the ED Parents Miranda Rights: Anything you say can and will be used against you by the eating disorder. You cannot, of course, control the way in which the sufferer will respond to what you say, and while it helps to be cautious, it doesn't help to constantly walk on eggshells. Here are the comments I found to be particularly harmful:

"You look like you're gaining weight quite nicely." To a person with an eating disorder, this means one thing and only one thing: You are getting fat. Instead, comment on their blossoming personality, the sparkle in their eyes, the bounce in their step. Stay away from comments on weight and shape. It's like walking through a field of land mines.

"I wish I had your problem." This completely invalidates the sufferer's experience, and can even fuel continued eating disordered behaviors. After all, if other people want to do what I'm doing, then it can't be that bad, right?

"Just eat!" Of course, if the person with an eating disorder is going to recover, they have to eat. But it's not as simple as "just" preparing a meal, "just" picking up a fork, and "just" eating. If the person with an eating disorder could eat normally, they would. They are scared. They can't "just" get over it—recovery takes lots of time and hard work.

"Think of all the people out there with *real* problems." Anorexia has a mortality rate of up to 20%. That sounds like a real problem to me. And comments like this may close down lines of communication between you and the sufferer because they might feel like you just don't understand.

"How can you think you're fat? You're a walking skeleton!" To a person with an eating disorder, distorted body image isn't distorted at all. The feelings of fatness are very intense and very real. You don't have to agree with them; you just have to believe. Support them. Ask how that makes them feel. Sympathize with how hard those feelings must be. And take the Fifth Amendment if they ask you if they look fat.

How to Approach a Loved One About Her Eating Disorder

Denial is much more than a river in Egypt—and more powerful, especially in a young person suffering from an eating disorder. Eating disorders are called *egosyntonic* by psychologists, which means that sufferers don't want to relinquish the disorder because they are accomplishing exactly what they set out to. Their pathological behaviors are having the right effects. What the sufferer might not be able to see are the effects that the eating disorder is having on them in other ways.

Educate yourself. If you suspect your loved one is suffering from an eating disorder, the best way to start is to learn more about the disorders. You can't find a solution unless you know more about the problem.

Pick a private time and place to approach the person. Confronting someone about an issue that is surrounded with secrecy and shame can bring up intense emotions for everyone involved. As well, privacy may allow the sufferer to be more candid and honest than if he or she were in a public place.

Don't overwhelm the person. This basically means that having 30 people in the room all talking about what they have observed will likely make the sufferer feel cornered. While you can bring up others' comments and concerns, it may be best to let other friends and family members talk to the sufferer at a different time and place.

It's also helpful to give your loved one plenty of time to respond to your concerns. Leave lots of time between comments and concerns. If caught off guard, it may take him time to articulate how he's feeling. By not interrupting or speaking too fast, it sends the message that you are truly listening.

Just the facts, ma'am. Rather than stating what you *suspect* is happening ("I don't think you're eating lunch at school."), say what you can confirm or see ("Your friends tell me that you throw away your lunch every day."). It's much harder for the sufferer to deny what's going on. Stick to the facts, and don't sound accusatory—the person is suffering from a disease.

Use "I" statements. I know this sounds a bit like psycho-babble, but it's also an effective way of communicating in any situation. Whatever the true situation actually is, it's hard to argue with your personal experience of your loved one's be-haviors. If you are worried about a particular behavior—say, continual trips to the bathroom after eating—then say some-thing along the lines of "When I see you run to the bathroom after meals, I get worried that you might be making yourself throw up. Can you talk to me about that?"

Expect denial. Especially in young adolescents, there is usu-ally a lot of confusion and very little insight to what is hap-pening. In the first stages of my eating disorder, I didn't think I had anorexia. I was just losing a little weight. I had no idea that you could lose too much weight. I didn't have a prob-lem—my parents were the ones with the problem, getting all worked up over something like this.

Another common diversionary tactic is for sufferers to turn the concern around to you. She may say that she's fine and it's *you* that is looking sickly or that has concerning habits. Thank her for the concern, and bring the conversation back around to your worries about her. You will deal with yourself, but right now, you need to deal with her situation.

Don't be afraid to seek help yourself. Dealing with a child with an eating disorder can be enormously stressful, and get-ting your own therapist, as well as meeting with your child's therapist and dietician, can help everyone get on the same page and give you peace of mind.

Remember, the earlier an eating disorder is diagnosed, the better the prognosis. Don't be afraid to speak up. Trust your instincts—odds are you know your child better than anyone.

Some Frequently Asked Questions for the Recently Diagnosed

Understanding Eating Disorders

I'm not underweight! How can I have an eating disorder?

An eating disorder has many other signs and symptoms (and causes of death) besides low bodyweight. If you suffer from anxiety surrounding food, spend much of your time thinking about what you are going to eat, how to avoid eating, planning your next binge and purge, and/or worrying about finding enough time to exercise, then you have a problem. Most people with eating disorders are of fairly normal weight. While the emaciated women and men featured on talk shows definitely suffer from anorexia nervosa, their appearance is not characteristic of the great majority of the eating disordered population, even those with anorexia.

My doctor has told me that I exercise too much. How can a person exercise too much?

For people with eating disorders, misusing exercise can be a form of purging unwanted calories. If you are not eating enough to meet your body's metabolic needs, you are much more prone to bone, ligament, and tendon damage. Your body needs time to heal between workouts. Many young female athletes suffer from the "female athlete triad": amenorrhea, osteoporosis, and eating disorders. It's okay to take a break from exercise, especially if you do not think that you can eat more to compensate for the increased activity. Wait and find an activity you love. Moving your body can be fun.

People tell me to "just eat!" or that I'm vain. Why won't people understand that it's so much more difficult than this?

A lot of the information spread around by popular media portrays people with eating disorders as rich, spoiled brats who are self-centered and obsessed with dieting. Any trip to an eating disorders clinic would, of course, disabuse them of this notion rather quickly. Obviously, in order to recover, you have to eat. But you wouldn't ask a person with cancer to "just kill all those cancer cells" and to "stop making such a big deal of things." Some people just won't understand and others aren't worth the effort. However, to those who really matter to you, providing some good books on the topic of eating disorders can go a long way to helping to improve their understanding.

Are "natural" dietary supplements and pills safe to take?

"Natural" does not necessarily mean "safe." Snake venom is natural. So is botulinum toxin, the most lethal substance known to man. Many herbal dietary supplements (including diet pills) are not regulated by the Food and Drug Administration (FDA) and therefore do not have to be proven both safe and effective. As a scientist, I choose not to purchase these substances unless they have been proven to be safe and effective in clinical trials. Also, they can interact with other medications you are taking, so be sure to tell your doctor all of the medication you are taking: prescription, over the counter, and herbal supplements.

I've just been diagnosed with an eating disorder, and I've been told that I will have it for the rest of my life. Do I have any hope to recover?

Absolutely! Research has shown that the great majority of young people diagnosed with an eating disorder do go on to recover and live happy, healthy, fulfilling lives. The road to recovery can be long and filled with plenty of ups and downs, but there is always hope. I hold onto that hope very closely. I believe firmly in complete recovery—it is my ultimate goal in life. I never want to forget that I had an eating disorder, because I know I have to remain vigilant about eating regularly, not overdoing the exercise, and taking my medications. However, that doesn't mean that I will be tormented by eating disorder thoughts.

Your best chances for a full recovery happen with early, intensive treatment. The sooner you reach a healthy weight and can stop binge eating and purging, the faster you will recover. These are not the only signs of recovery, but they are the most important steps. Your parents and treatment team can be an invaluable source of support during this time, and can help you regulate your eating and deal with the emotions that arise.

Getting Treatment

How do I know what type of treatment is best for me?

This is a question that is best discussed with your parents and your treatment team. They are the ones best qualified to make this decision. However, the question you asked has two parts: 1) the approach used in treatment and 2) the level of support you will need in order to fight the eating disorder. Some good questions to ask are:

- What are my immediate medical and psychiatric needs?
- Will I have the support to re-feed and/or stop binge eating and purging as an outpatient?
- Which eating disorder inpatient units or residential treatment centers are nearby?
- Will my insurance cover these treatments?
- What is the philosophy of my outpatient treatment team? Will that match up with the treatment I will receive if inpatient or residential treatment is necessary?
- What do my family and I think will work best for me?

There is no one right answer. I have used many different treatment modalities during my recovery process and have found all of them useful at various points in time. The most helpful *for me* were the behavioral therapies (CBT and DBT—see Chapter 4) that focused more on present issues and building skills to be effective in the world without the eating disorder.

How do I know if my therapist is right for me?

Psychotherapy is essentially a relationship between the therapist, you, and possibly your family. You may not click overnight—it takes time to build a trusting relationship. Give yourself a couple of visits if you remain unsure. Of course, if, at the end of the first session, you know the therapist isn't right for you, then feel free to move on. For me, I knew I had found the right therapist the moment I sat down with her. Dr. M., I learned, hated mornings and loved coffee. That, combined with other things, convinced me that I had found the right therapist for me—and I was right!

The best way to judge whether a therapist is right for you is based not only on your relationship and how comfortable you feel confiding in him/her, but also how well s/he is able to help you decrease and stop your eating disorder behaviors. I had a therapist who was sweet, and with whom I developed a good relationship, but my symptoms remained unchecked and eventually I was left with no choice but to seek out more intensive treatment.

What if my insurance won't cover the treatment that has been recommended to me by my treatment team? What can I do about this?

Ahhhh . . . insurance companies. Mental health coverage, and especially that for eating disorders, tends to, well, suck. Even in states with mental health parity (which means that the insurance companies are required by law to cover mental health illness on the same level as physical health illnesses), there have been denials of claims because anorexia and bulimia are not considered "biologically based mental illnesses." At the time this book went to press, there were several lawsuits pending that are challenging this very concept.

For now, you and your parents can talk with the insurance companies to negotiate coverage. It might not be much, but it's better than nothing. You are able to appeal any denial you receive, several times. Have your treatment team, as well as any treatment facility, advocate on your behalf. And most of all, document every interaction that goes on between you and the insurance company. Type up a document and print out one copy for your files and fax another to the insurance company. Their philosophy is: If it hasn't been documented, it didn't happen.

Lastly, you can pursue the matter legally, through a lawsuit. I'm not sue-happy, but should my insurance company deny my claims for my last round of residential treatment, I very well might take them to court over this matter. Because I don't want this happening to other people.

Until my insurance company agrees to cover my treatment, how will I pay?

You have several options. One is to pay out of pocket and pursue the insurance company later. This is, however, not always financially possible. Many therapists and dieticians have a sliding scale, and the fee is based on your family's ability to pay. This was a lifesaver for me during the time when I had no insurance coverage and a fairly low-paying job. Lastly, check with the United Way, any community mental health agencies, or your local public health department. Oftentimes, they know of free or very low-cost mental health services for people who can't otherwise afford them.

Moving Through Recovery

How am I supposed to recover when I don't feel ready?

This is one of the most common questions I get from sufferers. I told myself I would recover once I was "thin enough" or "sick enough." Other times, I wanted to wait to see that I was actually underweight before I would let myself start eating again. Mostly though, I was afraid of recovery. Afraid of failing, afraid of succeeding, afraid of life without the constant presence of the eating disorder.

Simply put, you will never feel ready to recover. The fear will not go away; ironically, it only seems to get worse the longer your eating disorder lasts. Your eating disorder will never let you feel thin enough or sick enough. I had to accept that last part, and it is still difficult, even after several years. I have no accurate perception of how sick I was. There are no prizes for the most ER visits in a week, no cards congratulating you for the lowest potassium level or for getting a feeding tube. My first step toward recovery was when I realized that I might not be ready to recover, but I was definitely ready to try something different.

I desperately want to recover, but I don't think I can. Other people can—I've seen it. But not me. Help!

Everyone recovers at their own pace, and everyone's recovery looks quite different. Sometimes, moving forward in recovery means you have to learn and develop new skills to be more effective in moving away from your eating disorder and in life in general. This takes time. You will get there. It helped me to remind myself that there was no good reason that I couldn't recover. I always thought I would never recover, never be able to eat without fear. And here I am, reassuring people about the very fears that I have overcome.

How am I supposed to eat and not purge when I feel so huge?

You can feel huge and still eat. This will not be pleasant. At all. But just because you are having difficulties with body image doesn't mean that you can't eat. It just makes it more challenging. The only way out is through. The best way to improve your body image is to maintain a healthy weight and stop other eating disorder behaviors. Realizing that my body image was distorted helped me, and can help you as well. I still saw myself as a whale when I looked in the mirror, but I reminded myself that things in the mirror are not always what they seem.

*I am working so hard at recovery, yet every time
I screw up and am right back at square one. Should I
even try anymore?*

Each time I slipped (and there were plenty of those!), I tried to
learn something from my experience, whether that was to treat
a bathroom scale like a nuclear device or to learn that it's much
more effective to reach out when I'm having thoughts of restricting rather than waiting until those behaviors have started.
The last time I entered treatment, I had been relapsing for over
one year before I finally came to the point that I could no longer
do it on my own. It was a brutal realization, but I have been in
strong recovery since.

You will likely fall on your butt as you recover from your
eating disorder. That's just the nature of recovery. But you will
never go back to square one. You are older and wiser, and have
learned new things along the way. Now you need to apply them.
Just remember the definition of insanity: doing the same thing
over and over and expecting different results.

Moving Out and Moving On

*I'm leaving for college soon. How do I cope with my
eating disorder while on campus?*

Judging from my own struggles with depression and OCD as
I went off to school, as well as information I've picked up from
others who have struggled with eating disorders during college,
the best way to prevent a resurgence of symptoms is to get to a
strong place in recovery before you enter school. College can be
a pressure cooker. I cracked a couple of times from the stress.
For me, the stress of college and the depression that followed

my return from a semester abroad was the straw that broke the camel's back.

That being said, college can be a fabulous, positive experience for many people, even those with eating disorders. There are several factors to evaluate as you consider the best way to deal with your eating disorder on campus. Here are some questions you may want to ask your college:

- What kind of counseling services do you offer for students? Are there community referrals?
- Is there a campus pharmacy? Do they take my insurance? Do they have the medications I need? If not, is there a pharmacy nearby that can provide these services for me?
- Do you have an eating disorder support group on campus? Is it facilitated by a recovered person or a professional? Are there any support groups in the community?
- How are the meals structured in the cafeteria? Do you offer a wide variety of foods for me to choose from?
- Is there a 24-hour number for me to call in a crisis?

Sadly, eating disorders are fairly common on most college campuses. You will not be alone in your struggles. While meeting other young adults with eating disorders can be a source of competition, it can also be a source of great support.

What else can I do to survive and enjoy my college and young adult life?

An eating disorder is a very isolating illness. Friendships can whither and die as your thoughts become increasingly focused on food and weight. People move on. Therefore, when you are starting recovery, you may be left with a limited support system. This has been one of the largest difficulties for me to overcome. I am a shy person by nature, and have a hard time meeting new people. So I started to join clubs in the community, such as a weekly knitting and crocheting get-together and an online book club, and took several classes through my local community education program.

It's also important to take proper care of all of your physical and emotional needs. I had to re-learn how to relax and have fun, that it was okay to watch TV and not do housework, or that taking a break didn't make me lazy or unproductive. There are many books and Web sites that have ideas for more positive ways to cope with stress, as well as to improve self-esteem and relationships.

Will I ever be able to have a normal life?

You will have the life that you choose for yourself. There are no guarantees. Like the t-shirt says: "Shit happens." But you always have the power to decide how you react to it. Remember, normal is just a setting on a washing machine. You can have a happy, fulfilling life after an eating disorder. Yes, an eating disorder can make life more challenging, but the journey of self-discovery on which you embark during recovery will often leave you wiser and more mature than your peers. These are gifts that will serve you no matter what path you choose in life.

Glossary

amenorrhea The absence of menstrual periods.

antidepressant A medication used to prevent or relieve depression.

antipsychotic A medication used to prevent or relieve psychotic symptoms. Some newer antipsychotics have mood-stabilizing effects as well.

anxiety disorder Any of several mental disorders that are characterized by extreme or maladaptive feelings of tension, fear, or worry.

atypical antipsychotic One of the newer antipsychotic medications. Some atypical antipsychotics are also used as mood stabilizers.

bipolar disorder A mood disorder characterized by an overly high mood, called mania, which alternates with depression. Also called manic depression.

body mass index (BMI) A measure of weight relative to height (calculated as weight in kilograms divided by height in meters squared. A calculator is available at http://www.nhlbisupport.com/bmi/).

cognitive-behavioral therapy (CBT) A form of psychotherapy that aims to correct ingrained patterns of thinking and behavior that may be contributing to a person's mental, emotional, or behavioral symptoms.

comorbidity The simultaneous presence of two or more disorders.

depression A feeling of being sad, hopeless, or apathetic that lasts for at least a couple of weeks. See **major depression**.

***Diagnostic and Statistical Manual of Mental Disorders*, Fourth Edition, Text Revision (DSM-IV)** A manual that mental health professionals use for diagnosing all kinds of mental illnesses.

dialectical-behavioral therapy (DBT) A form of psychotherapy that consists of four different modules: mindfulness, interpersonal effectiveness, distress tolerance, and emotion regulation.

eating disorder A disorder characterized by serious disturbances in eating behavior. People may severely restrict what they eat, or they may go on eating binges, then attempt to compensate by such means as self-induced vomiting or misuse of laxatives.

electrolytes   Salt constituents (sodium, potassium, chloride, and bicarbonate) found naturally in the bloodstream that are needed to maintain normal functions.

family therapy   Psychotherapy that brings together several members of a family for therapy sessions.

group therapy   Psychotherapy that brings together several patients with similar diagnoses or issues for therapy sessions.

hospitalization   Inpatient treatment in a facility that provides intensive, specialized care and close, round-the-clock monitoring.

individual therapy   Psychotherapy in which a patient meets one on one with a therapist.

interpersonal therapy (IPT)   A form of psychotherapy that aims to address the interpersonal triggers for mental, emotional, or behavioral symptoms.

laxative   A substance that helps promote bowel movements, that can be harmful and addicting if misused.

major depression   A mood disorder that involves either being depressed or irritable nearly all the time, or losing interest or enjoyment in almost everything. These feelings last for at least two weeks, are associated with several other symptoms, and cause significant distress or impaired functioning.

Maudsley method   A form of family therapy in which the parents actively participate in the recovery process, including overseeing meals.

menarche   The first occurrence of menstruation during puberty.

mental illness   A mental disorder that is characterized by abnormalities in mood, emotion, thought, or higher-order behaviors, such as social interaction or the planning of future activities.

mood   A pervasive emotion that colors a person's whole view of the world.

mood disorder   A mental disorder in which a disturbance in mood is the chief feature. Also called affective disorder.

mood stabilizer   A medication for bipolar disorder that reduces manic and/ or depressive symptoms and helps even out mood swings.

neurotransmitter   A chemical that acts as a messenger within the brain.

obsessive-compulsive disorder (OCD)   A mental disorder that is characterized by being obsessed with a certain idea and/or feeling compelled by an urgent need to engage in certain rituals.

partial hospitalization   Services such as individual and group therapy, special education, vocational training, parent counseling, and therapeutic recreational activities that are provided at least four hours per day.

perfectionism   A feeling that anything less than perfect is unacceptable.

personality disorder   A constellation of personality traits that significantly impair one's ability to function socially or that cause personal distress.

prevalence   The total number of cases of a disease existing in a given population at a given point in time or during a specified time.

psychiatrist   A medical doctor who specializes in the diagnosis and treatment of mental illnesses and emotional problems.

psychologist   A mental health professional who provides assessment and therapy for mental and emotional disorders. Also called a clinical psychologist.

psychosocial   Any situation in which both psychological and social factors are assumed to play a role.

psychotherapy   The treatment of a mental, emotional, or behavioral disorder through "talk therapy" and other psychological techniques.

purging   In the case of eating disorders, purging means to rid oneself of food eaten, either via chemically or self-induced vomiting or by using laxatives, diuretics, or enemas.

recurrence   A repeat episode of an illness.

relapse   The reemergence of symptoms after a period of remission.

remission   A return to the level of functioning that existed before an illness.

residential treatment center   A facility that provides round-the-clock supervision and care in a dorm-like group setting. The treatment is less specialized and intensive than in a hospital, but the length of stay is often considerably longer.

risk factor   A characteristic that increases a person's likelihood of developing an illness.

schizophrenia   A severe form of mental illness characterized by delusions, hallucinations, or serious disturbances in thought, behavior, or emotion.

selective serotonin reuptake inhibitor (SSRI)   A widely prescribed class of antidepressant.

serotonin   A neurotransmitter that plays a role in mood and helps regulate sleep, appetite, and sexual drive.

side effect   An unintended effect of a drug.

sociocultural   Involving both social and cultural factors.

substance abuse   The continued use of alcohol or other drugs despite negative consequences, such as dangerous behavior while under the influence or substance-related personal, social, or legal problems.

subtype   A group that is subordinate to a larger type or class.

suicidality   Suicidal thinking or behavior.

temperament   A person's inborn tendency to react to events in a particular way.

Resources

Organizations for Information and Support

All of the below organizations offer some type of information or support relating to eating disorders. Those marked with an asterisk (*) also have information on treatment providers and types of treatment.

Academy for Eating Disorders
60 Revere Drive, Suite 500
Northbrook, IL 60062-1577
(847) 498-4274
www.aedweb.org

Alliance for Eating Disorders Awareness
PO Box 13155
North Palm Beach, FL 33408-3155
(866) 662-1235
www.eatingdisorderinfo.org

American Academy of Pediatrics (AAP)
141 Northwest Point Blvd.
Elk Grove Village, IL 60007-1098
(847) 434-4000
www.aap.org

*American Dietetic Association
120 South Riverside Plaza, Suite 2000
Chicago, IL 60606-6995

(800) 877-1600
www.eatright.org

Anorexia Nervosa and Related Eating Disorders (ANRED)
603 Stewart St.
Seattle, WA 98101
(800) 931-2237
www.anred.com

Bazelon Center for Mental Health Law
1101 15th St., NW, Suite 1212
Washington, DC 20005
(202) 467-5730
www.bazelon.org

Center for Young Women's Health
Children's Hospital Boston
333 Longwood Ave., 5th floor
Boston, MA 02115
(617) 355-2994
www.youngwomenshealth.org

Eating Disorders Association (EDA)
103 Prince of Wales Rd.
Norwich NR1 1DW
United Kingdom
0870-770-3256
www.b-eat.co.uk/Home

*Eating Disorder Referral and Information Center
2923 Sandy Pointe, Suite 6
Del Mar, CA 92014-2052
858-481-1515
www.edreferral.com

Eating Disorders Coalition
611 Pennsylvania Ave., SE, 423
Washington, DC 20003-4303
(202) 543-9570
www.eatingdisorderscoalition.org

*Gurze Books Eating Disorders Resources
PO Box 2238
Carlsbad, CA 92018

(800) 756-7533
www.gurze.com

Harris Center for Education and Advocacy in Eating Disorders
2 Long Fellow Pl., Suite 200
Boston, MA 02114
(617) 726-8470
www.harriscentermgh.org

International Association of Eating Disorders Professionals
PO Box 1295
Pekin, IL 61555
(800) 800-8126
www.iaedp.com

Lifelines Foundation for Eating Disorders
10304 Buffalo Ridge
Waco, TX 76712
(254) 420-3947
www.lfed.org

*National Association of Anorexia Nervosa and Associated Disorders (ANAD)
PO Box 7
Highland Park, IL 60035
(847) 831-3438
www.anad.org
(also sponsors free support groups)

*National Eating Disorders Association (NEDA)
603 Stewart St., Suite 803
Seattle, WA 98101
(206) 382-3587
www.nationaleatingdisorders.org

National Eating Disorder Information Centre-Canada (NEDIC)
ES 7-421, 200 Elizabeth St.
Toronto, Canada M5G 2C4
(866) 633-4230 (toll free in Canada)
(416) 340-4156
www.nedic.ca

*Something Fishy Web site on Eating Disorders
www.something-fishy.org
(also has moderated recovery support bulletin boards)

Books

Some of the books mentioned below may be challenging to read and may contain material that could be triggering. Although I believe that they are ultimately worth the read, please use your best judgment in determining whether or not a book would be appropriate for you.

Bordo, Susan. *Unbearable Weight: Feminism, Western Culture, and the Body.* Berkeley, CA: University of California Press, 1995.

Brumberg, Joan Jacobs. *Fasting Girls: The History of Anorexia Nervosa.* New York: Vintage Books, 2000.

———. *The Body Project: An Intimate History of American Girls.* New York: Vintage Books, 1998.

Gordon, Richard. *Eating Disorders: Anatomy of a Social Epidemic.* 2nd ed. Oxford, UK: Blackwell Publishers, 2000.

Hall, Lindsey and Leigh Cohn. *Bulimia: A Guide to Recovery.* Carlsbad, CA: Gurze Books, 1998.

Hall, Lindsey and Monika Ostroff. *Anorexia Nervosa: A Guide to Recovery.* Carlsbad, CA: Gurze Books, 1999.

Hesse-Biber, Sharlene. *Am I Thin Enough Yet?: The Cult of Thinness and the Commercialization of Identity.* New York: Oxford University Press, 1996.

Johnson, Anita. *Eating in the Light of the Moon: How Women Can Transform Their Relationship With Food Through Myths, Metaphors, and Storytelling.* Carlsbad, CA: Gurze Books, 2000.

Roth, Geneen. *When You Eat at the Refrigerator, Pull Up a Chair.* New York: Hyperion, 1998.

Sacker, Ira M. and Mark A. Zimmer. *Dying to Be Thin: Understanding and Defeating Anorexia Nervosa and Bulimia—A Practical, Lifesaving Guide.* New York: Warner Books, 1987.

Wolf, Naomi. *The Beauty Myth: How Images of Beauty Are Used Against Women.* New York: Anchor Books, 1992.

First-Person Accounts

Arnold, Carrie. *Running on Empty: A Diary of Anorexia and Recovery.* Livonia, MI: First Page Publications, 2004.

Edut, Ophira and Rebecca Walker, eds. *Body Outlaws: Rewriting the Rules of Beauty and Body Image.* Seattle: Seal Press, 2000.

Hall, Lindsey. *Full Lives: Women Who Have Freed Themselves From the Food and Weight Obsession.* Carlsbad, CA: Gurze Books, 1993.

Knapp, Carolyn. *Appetites: Why Women Want.* New York: Counterpoint Press, 2003.

Lerner, Betsy. *Food and Loathing: A Lament.* New York: Simon and Schuster, 2003.

Rhodes, Constance. *Life Inside the "Thin" Cage: A Personal Look Into the Hidden World of the Chronic Dieter.* New York: Shaw Books, 2003.

Schaeffer, Jenni (with Thom Rutledge). *Life Without Ed: How One Woman Declared Independence from Her Eating Disorder and How You Can Too.* New York: McGraw-Hill, 2004.

Shanker, Wendy. *The Fat Girl's Guide to Life.* New York: Bloomsbury USA, 2004.

Help for Related Mental Health Issues

General Information

National Institutes of Mental Health, (866) 615-6464, www.nimh.nih.gov

American Academy of Child and Adolescent Psychiatry, (202) 966-7300, www.aacap.org, www.parentsmedguide.org

American Psychiatric Association, (888) 357-7924, www.psych.org, www.healthy minds.org

American Psychological Association, (800) 374-2721, www.apa.org, www.apahelpcenter.org

Mood Disorders

ORGANIZATIONS

American Association of Suicidology, (202) 237-2280, www.suicidology.org

American Foundation for Suicide Prevention, (888) 333-2377, www.afsp.org

Depression and Bipolar Support Alliance, (800) 826-3632, www.dbsalliance.org

Depression and Related Affective Disorders Association, (410) 583-2919, www.drada.org

National Alliance on Mental Illness, (800) 950–6264, www.nami.org

BOOKS

Irwin, Cait, with Dwight L. Evans and Linda Wasmer Andrews. *Monochrome Days: A Firsthand Account of One Teenager's Experience With Depression.* New York: Oxford University Press with the Annenberg Foundation Trust at Sunnylands and the Annenberg Public Policy Center at the University of Pennsylvania, 2007.

Jamison, Kay Redfield. *Night Falls Fast: Understanding Suicide.* New York: Vintage, 2000.

Jamieson, Patrick E., with Moira A. Rynn. *Mind Race: A Firsthand Account of One Teenager's Experience With Bipolar Disorder.* New York: Oxford University Press with the Annenberg Foundation Trust at Sunnylands and the Annenberg Public Policy Center at the University of Pennsylvania, 2006.

Solomon, Andrew. *The Noonday Demon: An Atlas of Depression.* New York: Scribner, 2001.

Web Sites

MindZone, Annenberg Foundation Trust at Sunnylands with the Annenberg
   Public Policy Center of the University of Pennsylvania, www.CopeCareDeal.org
TeensHealth, Nemours Foundation, www.teenshealth.org

Anxiety Disorders

Organizations

Anxiety Disorders Association of America, (240) 485-1001, www.adaa.org
Obsessive Compulsive Foundation, (203) 401-2070, www.ocfoundation.org

Books

Ford, Emily, with Michael Liebowitz, M.D., and Linda Wasmer Andrews. *What
   You Must Think of Me: A Firsthand Account of One Teenager's Experience with
   Social Anxiety Disorder.* New York: Oxford University Press with the Annenberg
   Foundation Trust at Sunnylands and the Annenberg Public Policy Center at the
   University of Pennsylvania, 2007.
Kant, Jared Douglas, with Martin Franklin, Ph.D., and Linda Wasmer Andrews.
   *The Thought That Counts: A Firsthand Account of One Teenager's Experience With
   Obsessive-Compulsive Disorder.* New York: Oxford University Press with the
   Annenberg Foundation Trust at Sunnylands and the Annenberg Public Policy
   Center at the University of Pennsylvania, forthcoming in 2008.
Marra, Thomas. *Depressed and Anxious.* Oakland, CA: New Harbinger Publica-
   tions, 2004.
Schwartz, Jeffrey. *Brain Lock: Free Yourself from Obsessive-Compulsive Behavior.*
   New York: Regan Books, 1997.

Web Sites

Freedom from Fear, www.freedomfromfear.org

Substance Abuse

Organizations

Alcoholics Anonymous, (212) 870-3400 (check your phone book for a local
   number), www.aa.org
American Council for Drug Education, (800) 488-3784, www.acde.org
Narcotics Anonymous, (818) 773-9999, www.na.org
National Council on Alcoholism and Drug Dependence, (800) 622-2255,
   www.ncadd.org
National Institute on Alcohol Abuse and Alcoholism, (301) 443-3860,
   www.niaaa.nih.gov, www.collegedrinkingprevention.gov

National Institute on Drug Abuse, (301) 443-1124, www.drugabuse.gov, teens.drugabuse.gov

Partnership for a Drug-Free America, (212) 922-1560, www.drugfreeamerica.com

Substance Abuse and Mental Health Services Administration, (800) 729–6686, ncadi.samhsa.gov, csat.samhsa.gov, prevention.samhsa.gov

BOOK

Keegan, Kyle, with Howard B. Moss, M.D., and Beryl Lieff Benderly. *Chasing the High: A Firsthand Account of One Young Person's Experience With Substance Abuse.* New York: Oxford University Press with the Annenberg Foundation Trust at Sunnylands and the Annenberg Public Policy Center at the University of Pennsylvania, forthcoming in 2008.

WEB SITES

Facts on Tap, Phoenix House, www.factsontap.org

Freevibe, National Youth Anti-Drug Media Campaign, www.freevibe.com

The New Science of Addiction: Genetics and the Brain, Genetic Science Learning Center at the University of Utah, learn.genetics.utah.edu/units/addiction

Self-Injury

ORGANIZATIONS

American Self-Harm Information Clearinghouse, www.selfinjury.org

BOOKS

Alderman, Tracy. *The Scarred Soul: Understanding and Ending Self-Inflicted Violence.* Oakland, CA: New Harbinger Publications, 1997.

Kingsonbloom, Jennifer, Karen Conterio, and Wendy Lader. *Bodily Harm: The Breakthrough Program for Self-Injurers.* New York: Hyperion, 1999.

Lezine, DeQuincy A., Ph.D., with David Brent, M.D. *Eight Stories Up: An Adolescent Chooses Hope Over Suicide.* New York: Oxford University Press with the Annenberg Foundation Trust at Sunnylands and the Annenberg Public Policy Center at the University of Pennsylvania, forthcoming in 2008.

WEB SITES

Self-Abuse Finally Ends (SAFE Alternatives), www.selfinjury.com

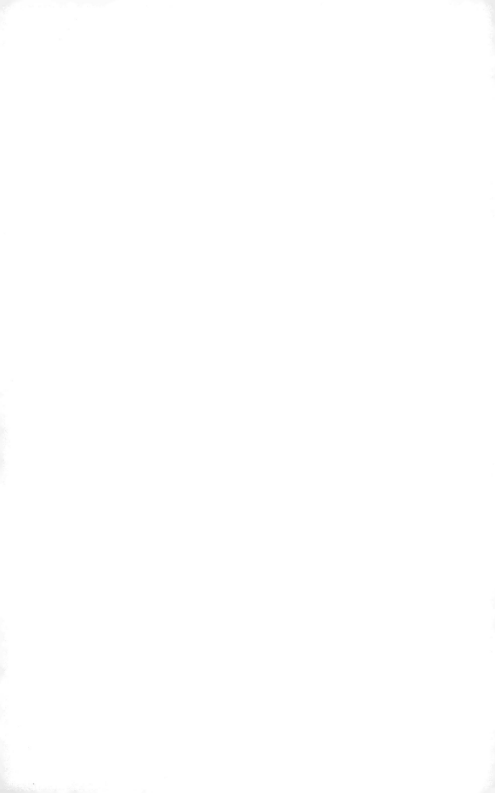

Bibliography

Abuse "triggers eating disorders." BBC Health News, November 9, 2005. http://
news.bbc.co.uk/1/hi/health/4417938.stm. Accessed 12/21/06.

American Academy of Pediatrics Committee on Adolescence. Identifying and
treating eating disorders. *Pediatrics* 111 (2003): 204–211. http://aappolicy.
aappublications.org/cgi/content/full/pediatrics, 111/1/204. Accessed 12/21/06.

American Psychiatric Association. *Diagnostic and Statistical Manual of Mental
Disorders* (4th ed., text revision). Washington, DC: American Psychiatric Association, 2000.

Bacanu, S. M., et al. Linkage analysis of anorexia and bulimia nervosa cohorts using
selected behavioral phenotypes as quantitative traits or covariates. *American
Journal of Medical Genetics Part B: Neuropsychiatric Genetics* 139B:1 (2005):
61–68.

Bailer U. F., et al. Altered brain serotonin 5-HT1A receptor binding after recovery
from anorexia nervosa measured by positron emission tomography and
[carbonyl11C]WAY-100635. *Archives of General Psychiatry* 62:9 (2005):
1032–41.

Bennett, Jessica. Unrealistic weights. *Newsweek* (November 15, 2006). www.msnbc.
msn.com/ id/15730915/site/newsweek/. Accessed 12/21/06.

Borderline Personality Disorder. *NIMH: NIH Publication No. 01–4938.* 2001.
www.nimh.nih.gov/publicat/bpd.cfm. Accessed 11/13/06.

Evans, Dwight L., and Linda Wasmer Andrews. *If Your Adolescent Has Depression or
Bipolar Disorder: An Essential Resource for Parents.* New York: Oxford University
Press with the Annenberg Foundation Trust at Sunnylands and the Annenberg
Public Policy Center at the University of Pennsylvania, 2005.

Evans, Dwight L., Edna B. Foa, Raquel E. Gur, Herbert Hendin, Charles P.
O'Brien, Martin E.P. Seligman, and B. Timothy Walsh. *Treating and
Preventing Adolescent Mental Health Disorders: What We Know and What We*

Don't Know—A Research Agenda for Improving the Mental Health of Our Youth. New York: Oxford University Press with the Annenberg Foundation Trust at Sunnylands and the Annenberg Public Policy Center at the University of Pennsylvania, 2005.

Hatch, K. A., et al. An objective means of diagnosing anorexia nervosa and bulimia nervosa using $(15)N/(14)N$ and $(13)C/(12)C$ ratios in hair. *Rapid Communications in Mass Spectrometry* 20:22 (2006): 3367–3373.

Irwin, Cait, with Dwight L. Evans and Linda Wasmer Andrews. *Monochrome Days: A Firsthand Account of One Teenager's Experience with Depression.* New York: Oxford University Press with the Annenberg Foundation Trust at Sunnylands and the Annenberg Public Policy Center at the University of Pennsylvania, 2007.

Jamieson, Patrick, with Moira Rynn. *Mind Race: A Firsthand Account of One Teenager's Experience with Bipolar Disorder.* New York: Oxford University Press with the Annenberg Foundation Trust at Sunnylands and the Annenberg Public Policy Center at the University of Pennsylvania, 2006.

Johnson, Carla K. Reading diet articles could be unhealthy. Newsreview.info, January 2, 2007. http://hosted.ap.org/dynamic/stories/D/DIET_GIRLS_MAG AZINES?SITE=ORROS&SECTION=HOME&TEMPLATE=DEFAULT#. Accessed 1/04/07.

Johnson, Craig. Speech given at the Renfrew Center Foundation Conference, "Feminist Perspectives on Eating Disorders: Enduring Wisdom, New Frontiers." Philadelphia, PA, November 14, 2005.

Levitan, R. D., et al. The serotonin-1Dbeta receptor gene and severity of obsessive-compulsive disorder in women with bulimia nervosa. *European Neuropsychopharmacology* 16:1 (2006): 1–6.

Lucas, Alexander R. *Demystifying Anorexia Nervosa: An Optimistic Guide to Understanding and Healing.* New York: Oxford University Press, 2004.

Taylor C. B., et al. Prevention of eating disorders in at-risk college-age women. *Archives of General Psychiatry* 63:8 (2006): 881–8.

Walsh B. T. "Two Hot Topics: Psychopharmacology and DSM-V." National Eating Disorders Association Conference, September. 15, 2006.

Walsh B. T., et al. Fluoxetine after weight restoration in anorexia nervosa: a randomized control trial. *JAMA* 295:22 (2006): 2605–2612.

Walsh, B. Timothy, and V. L. Cameron. *If Your Adolescent Has an Eating Disorder: An Essential Resource for Parents.* New York: Oxford University Press with the Annenberg Foundation Trust at Sunnylands and the Annenberg Public Policy Center at the University of Pennsylvania, 2005.

Zerbe, Katherine. *The Body Betrayed: A Deeper Understanding of Women, Eating Disorders, and Treatment.* Carlsbad: Gurze Books, 1995.

Index

AAP. *See* American Academy of Pediatrics
Academy for Eating Disorders, 151
Acceptance of illness, 9–11, 85. *See also* Realization of illness
Activities, social
 recovery through, 70, 73, 88, 89–90, 109, 145–46
 risk factors associated to, 43
Advocacy, 130–31
Affirmations, 92–93
AIDS, 14–15, 22, 105
Alliance for Eating Disorders Awareness, 151
Amenorrhea, 47
American Academy of Child and Adolescent Psychiatry, Web site for, 76
American Academy of Pediatrics (AAP), 151
American Dietetic Association, 61, 151–52
ANAD. *See* National Association of Anorexia Nervosa and Associated Disorders

AN-BP. *See* Anorexia nervosa binge eating/purging
Anemia, 48
Animal therapy, 91
Annenberg Foundation Trust, xiv
Anorexia nervosa. *See also* Eating disorder(s); Risk factors, eating disorder
 activities/sports related to, 43
 ages associated with, 36
 anxiety's relation to, 18–20, 30, 36, 38, 51–52
 brain chemistry's relation to, 36, 37, 45
 diagnostic migration and, 53
 disorders co-occurring with, 8, 12, 14–15, 18–20, 24, 49–53
 gender statistics on, 28
 genetic predisposition toward, 37, 45
 history of, 34
 medication for treatment of, 45–46, 74–75, 121
 occurrence statistics on, 28
 personality traits associated with, 13–14, 30, 37–39, 45